AUTOBIOGRAPHY
of a
SEA CREATURE

Perspectives in Health Humanities

UC Health Humanities Press publishes scholarship produced or reviewed under the auspices of the University of California Health Humanities Consortium, a multi-campus collaborative of faculty, students, and trainees in the humanities, medicine, and health sciences. Our series invites scholars from the humanities and health care professions to share narratives and analysis on health, healing, and the contexts of our beliefs and practices that impact biomedical inquiry.

General Editor

Brian Dolan, PhD, Professor, Department of Humanities and Social Sciences, University of California, San Francisco (UCSF)

Other Titles in this Series

Heart Murmurs: What Patients Teach Their Doctors
Edited by Sharon Dobie, MD (2014)

Humanitas: Readings in the Development of the Medical Humanities
Edited by Brian Dolan (2015)

Follow the Money: Funding Research in a Large Academic Health Center
Henry R. Bourne and Eric B. Vermillion (2016)

Soul Stories: Voices from the Margins
Josephine Ensign (2018)

Fixing Women: The Birth of Obstetrics and Gynecology in Britain and America
Marcia D. Nichols (2021)

www.UCHealthHumanitiesPress.com

This series is made possible by the generous support of the Dean of the School of Medicine at UCSF, the UCSF Library, and a Multicampus Research Program Grant from the University of California Office of the President. Grant ID MR-15-328363 and Grant ID M23PR5992.

AUTOBIOGRAPHY
of a
SEA CREATURE

~

Healing the Trauma of Infant Surgery

WENDY PATRICE WILLIAMS

University of California
Center for Health Humanities
Department of Humanities and Social Sciences
UCSF (Box 0850)
490 Illinois Street, Floor 7
San Francisco, CA 94143-0850

Cover image used courtesy of the artist.
Ronda Waiksnis, *Post Rain, Rough Water*, Abstract Oil Painting on Arches paper. Height: 22 in (55.88 cm) Width: 30 in (76.2 cm) Depth: 0.1 in (2.54 mm) (2020) Artist's comments: Abstracted view of a clearing storm. Moody black and navy clouds give way to a pale sunset in the distance. "Nature's colors are represented here in full visceral fashion."
For more information: https://www.rwaiksnis.com/biography

Production design by Virtuoso Press

Library of Congress Control Number: 2023935491

ISBN: 978-1-7355423-5-5

Printed in USA

"In this absorbing book, we are privileged to join Wendy in her journey of 50 years to recover from surgery as an infant when anesthesia was not routinely administered. Ironically, this life-saving operation resulted in the question she could not address with certainty until she was 52 – was she dead or alive? You will be riveted by the chronicling of her experiences and the way she weaves together her inside and outside life as she uses creative processes – breath work, drawings, journaling, and the exploration of her powerful dreams – to search for the answer. Like her role model the biologist Rachel Carson, Wendy crafts exquisite observations of the natural world and her beloved sea creatures, sprinkled like tiny jewels throughout her writing. Reading this book will send you on a most memorable odyssey into a child's world that few people have been able to make."

— *Dr. Linda Gantt*, PhD, ATR-BC, is the owner and Executive Director of Intensive Trauma Recovery and ITR Training Institute LLC. In late 2020, she co-founded Help For Trauma Inc., a non-profit established to fund trauma research and offer trauma-effective training to mental health workers.

"In *Autobiography of a Sea Creature*, Wendy gives a voice to infants unable to articulate, who, due to necessary medical procedures, experience trauma. We journey with Wendy as she discovers the profound physical and emotional effects of this initial surgery and its consequences throughout her life. She shows us that the tentacles of the trauma extend and blend beyond her to her family and relationships. With the sea and its creatures interwoven in her life, the reader can also ride the fluid waves into healing and well being. With the growing awareness of trauma and PTSD in the world, this autobiography is one of support for both our precious little ones and all adults who were infants at one time."

— *Jean Anne Zollars*, PT, DPT, MA, BI-D, Instructor in Visceral and Neural Manipulation for the Barral Institute, specializing in Pediatrics. Upcoming book: *Visceral Manipulation for Pediatrics*. www.jazollarspt.com

"*Autobiography of a Sea Creature* is not just a story of one woman's emotional and psychological rebirth from the trauma of infant surgery. It is the poetic, haunting, life-affirming journey of healing an ecosystem, whether that is our human body or our planet. Wendy Williams has written an evocative memoir of awakening that will inspire anyone who cares about resilience, self-exploration, and our capacity for compassion."

— *Mary Fifield*
Fire & Water: Stories from the Anthropocene
Available now: https://www.fireandwaterstories.com/

This book is dedicated to

Lee O. Johnson, the therapist who first validated my emotional suffering

from early surgery;

psychiatrist Dr. Louis Tinnin, who, along with Dr. Linda Gantt, founded

Intensive Trauma Therapy, Inc., a clinic which helped many survivors of

infant surgery without anesthesia or adequate pain control;

and to all the precious sea creatures everywhere.

Author's Note: The names and identifying characteristics of some people have been changed to protect their privacy.

Contents

Foreword

by Fred L. Vanderbom

It was on a quiet Sunday afternoon in February 2009 when I found a freshly uploaded post by an American woman who wrote about how the horseshoe crabs on a beach linked her to her emotional struggles with the effects of her infant surgery for pyloric stenosis. Wendy Williams and I started a correspondence and a partnership in both discovery and blogging that have taught and affirmed each of us in our deep hunger to understand the emotions that arose from our early surgeries and which have left us with degrees of PTSD.

Many pre-1990s babies who had infant surgery were affected by the long-held belief that "babies don't feel or remember pain." A range of methods, from risky total anesthesia to paralyzing drugs, was used to prevent writhing and shrieking in pain during surgical procedures, be they circumcisions or heart operations. A landmark study by Drs. K. J. S. Anand and P. R. Hickey, published in the November 1987 *New England Journal of Medicine*, led to a rapid and complete change in attitude and protocols.

At about the same time, a growing interest in the effects of early and pre-verbal trauma on babies and infants revealed that trauma that is not consciously remembered can seriously affect these people in later life. It was the recognition of "somatic" (body as opposed to mind) memory that prompted Wendy, me, and many others to explore what might be causing some of the mystery symptoms of our formative and later years. This search brought me to Wendy's first post, just minutes after it had been uploaded.

Although both of us are wordsmiths, Wendy's blogging journey

(ReStoryyourlife.com) was different from mine in several respects. She has been more inquisitive and assertive, and being American she has had access to a much bigger "market" than I have: many more trauma survivors, professionals, and support organizations. She has built up and benefited from self-help and healing therapies and identified many books, speakers, and writers who have added to our joint pool of knowledge.

Through most of the intervening years, Wendy has written up her journey with a view to publishing it to reach an even wider readership than her blogging and personal advocacy could ever do. I read the draft manuscript some years ago and am thrilled that the finished book is now in your hands. She has written not so much to tell her story as to share the rich pool of knowledge and resources she has gathered.

Everyone affected by trauma experiences this in their own way, but the related events, reactions, and help have many common threads. Wendy's story and self-discoveries will add light to everyone possibly affected by or interested in pre-1990s early infant surgery.

Fred L. Vanderbom
https://survivinginfantsurgery.wordpress.com/
Adelaide, South Australia

i asked my mentor

in our happy hours

the ins and outs of this life

and far beyond

he said

our salvation is on the way

when you try to take

people's pain away.

—*Rumi*, translated by Nader Khalili

Depression, I now believe, is linked to a complex story not yet written.

—Louise de Salvo

Prologue

The nurse dabbed my arm with a wet cotton ball and pricked me with a needle. Dr. Constad's voice was warm gravel. "Look at you," he said, squatting so his eyes were at equal height with mine. "You are a miracle." Happiness filled up my little body, like air rushing into a balloon, and I looked at my mother who stood anxiously beside me. "Unbelievable," he continued. "I wouldn't have bet a plug nickel on you when you were a baby." The balloon burst. I was so ashamed I could hardly hear him continue, "but look at you now."

As soon as I was naked on the examining table, his hands kneaded my stomach. He dug deep, asking questions with his fingertips and palms. I stared at the ceiling, afraid. He searched quickly, furiously, but methodically, bent on discovering something hard, that olive of stone, seed of death. His hands seemed determined to find any possible intruder.

"I don't feel anything hard," Dr. Constad pronounced. "Nice and soft."

"Will she have trouble with her stomach later, say when she's fifty?"

"She shouldn't. We'll keep checking, of course."

I had no idea what fifty meant. I was not yet two when I started to worry.

Horseshoe Crabs

There is no such thing as a routine operation in a baby.

—Catherine Musemeche, MD,
pediatric surgeon, author of *Small*

The day after I was admitted to the hospital, my mother waited near a single sterile room where the nurses would bring me after surgery. She had arrived early to the ward, after sending Dad to work and my brother, Wayne, to Aunt Terry's, only to find that her twenty-six-day old infant had been whisked away to surgery hours earlier. I was failing, the staff told her—no time for signing consents.

That was the darkest hour of her life. She paced the hallway, stood at the window and watched people below, rushing by on Chancellor Avenue. She wanted to be one of them with regular cares. She remembers every thought as if her mind were a movie camera.

After the operation, the nurses wheeled me into a hospital room made of glass. They did not speak to my mother as she stood in the hallway and waited while they settled me. No one ever came back out to offer a word of support or explain how the operation went. I was laid into a crib enclosed by an oxygen tent and pushed near the observation window so my mother could see me from the hallway.

"A tiny lump wrapped in black hoses, the diameter of a quarter," my mother always said. "You looked like an alien. Even so, I wished I could pick you up and hold you, but I wasn't allowed in. Besides, you were too fragile, the tubes too big."

The nurses injected me with food with something that looked like a large syringe. Day and night, the nurses observed me through a large window. My mother made sure she was beside me at her window every morning at six a.m. She'd wake up and be frightened by that empty crib beside her. When there's a crib at home without a baby in it, that baby is at death's door.

I had a condition called pyloric stenosis. The muscle around the pyloric valve between the stomach and small intestine swelled and food could not pass through. This problem is more easily diagnosed nowadays and the remedy less severe, but in 1952, the obstetrician diagnosed my symptoms incorrectly and by the time I had surgery to open the passageway at twenty-six days old, I weighed only four pounds, down from six pounds, seven ounces.

I used to believe that my mother saved my life single-handedly. Her stories said as much. I pictured her as twice her size, bent over a huge medical book propped up on a lectern at the public library as she searched day after day for the cause of my illness, flipping page after page, then suddenly pointing to the obscure paragraph describing my symptoms: *projectile vomiting, weight loss.* "Pyloric stenosis!" she cried. To me, she was Supermom. A God, only more so: she gave me life twice.

In fact, it was like I had two birthdays: the official one July 1, 1952 and the unofficial one July 26, 1952 that only my mother and I recognized—the date of my operation. My mother says that she thinks of that second one as "my christening." All my life, on my unofficial birthday, she said to me, "Do you know what day this is?" and I always answered, "Yes." Then she set the needle in the groove and played that same old song: *There were tubes everywhere, in and out of every opening. Tubes even coming out of your head. You looked like an alien from outer space!* There were variations but essentially, the same tune year in and year out.

Dr. Constad, my brother's pediatrician, actually saved my life by looking in on me during a house visit for Wayne. I was less than a month old and was obviously failing to thrive. The light drained from his face, my mother told me, when he saw me in my crib. "Take her to the hospital immediately," he said.

Dead babies haunted our family. Francis Albert, my mother's brother, died of a high fever at three years old. Her cousins, four infant boys, died of what was then called "summer's complaint" and later understood to be lactose intolerance. The row of small white gravestones are smooth now, the words long rubbed away. Wayne was very sick as a baby. Somehow, as my mother tells the story, he was exposed to radiator fluid after she gave birth to him in the back seat of their car where my father had piled old rusty radiators. Wayne recovered in an incubator. A few years later, doctors thought he had leukemia and hospitalized him. Tests revealed that he was allergic to cow's milk. Two premature babies of my mother's died ten years before Wayne was born, one came during a hurricane and the other as the result of a car accident. Dead babies. Dead babies everywhere.

My mother used to tell me that back in the old days, dead babies were not buried in their own plots but placed in caskets with anonymous adults. I imagined a dead baby lying on the chest of a corpse and oddly sensed the weight of this baby on my chest each night before bed, my breath shallow. I had come to think of it as a giant moth wrapped up, like a mummy, as though a spider had seized her—a dead baby wound round in bandages, bound by tubes like spaghetti red with tomato sauce, roping in and out of every opening like worms. *You looked like an alien being, a creature from outer space*—my mother's words, the way she described me hundreds of times during my life. Not even a baby, dead or alive.

Once I dreamed that my mother and I stared into a toilet at what looked like a slab of meat in the bowl. What to do with it, we wondered.

"Stuff it down," my mother said, "it'll go."

"It'll clog the pipes," I said. "It won't fit."

My mother flushed anyway. The bowl filled with churning water and overflowed. It wouldn't go down, but she kept trying.

In records from my hospitalization after my suicide attempt at age twenty-two, I found the familiar phrase *26 days old*. My mother had told the social worker about the operation that I had undergone as an infant; he wrote no special note to follow up on this information. The report focused on my thyroid gland and the irregularity of my periods. Blood had been drawn, a gynecology exam administered—hormones, or female problems, were apparently key in my admittance to the hospital.

The notes refer to a brief meeting with the psychiatrist, his prescription for anti-depressants, and to a consultation with a social worker three weeks after my admission: *Patient advised to seek employment (want ads given to patient). Patient should pursue stable family life (stipend allotted for purchase of feminine hygiene products and new clothes).*

My cold turkey withdrawal from Valium prescribed for tension and pain in my jaw—the actual precipitating factor of my breakdown—was not something worth mentioning. A prescription for Valium was thought of like aspirin at that time: Take it 4 times a day and whenever needed to relieve the pain.

Years later, with the encouragement of my therapist, I drew the image I had of myself as a baby—a floating monster, wound round with strands of red spaghetti. A fetal body with a blue belly and blue rubbery legs, small feet webbed like a duck's. Bald, blue head and red face. Giant amber insect eyes as if on fire, the eyes windows to my insides. A gash on my belly, red and purple angry strokes. In the picture, my hands are huge, held up as if screaming, *STOP!* Yet the fingers are limp, wavy as if boneless. In fact my whole body is floppy, cast adrift, given up as if flowing with a current.

I carried this image of my beginnings—a larval creature floating in outer space. A baby who, in all likelihood, had not received anesthesia for stomach surgery at four weeks old and was given a muscle paralyzer so that she could not fight. A baby who was awake. At the time, it was believed that anesthetic drugs were too dangerous for infants. Besides, they rationalized, babies did not feel pain. And if they did, they would not remember.

There were tubes everywhere, in and out of every opening. —Mother

I began to gain weight. The surgeon met with my mother when I was ready to go home from the hospital. I was just under two months old. He told her in what my mother called "thick German," that my survival hinged on her ability to keep me from crying. "Mrs. Villiams," he said, "vee vill not be doing surgery again." There were two sets of stitches, she understood, one around the pylorus valve, between the stomach and small intestine, and a second set closing my abdomen. If I cried, he explained, the stitches would burst and I would die.

My mother was grim. That night she huddled with my father, and they drew up a battle plan. During the day while he was at work, she would stand watch, picking me up the second I started crying. In the evening, my father would stand guard while she cooked and cleaned up. The war was on. They worked together to keep me from crying and neglected my three-year-old brother, Wayne.

My mother and my dad worked as a team. On weekends, they put me out in a bassinet in front of the fireplace for visitors to see.

I had a distinctive way of crying, a kind of subdued whimper, and Wayne learned it. When company sat around the living room, oohing and ahhing over me in the bassinet, Wayne stood in the middle of the room, imitating my cries—"hew, hew"—his face screwed up with fake tears. Mom thought it the oddest thing.

Each morning, during those early days after I arrived home from the hospital, my three-year-old brother headed for the street corner and kicked the curb near the sewer. Just kicked and kicked. When Dr. Constad arrived for a home visit to check me, he asked my mother why Wayne was sitting alone on the curb down the street. She told him that she was so busy caring for me, she had no time for him. "If you don't pay that poor kid some attention, he's going to grow up with a huge hatred." The doctor's observation confirmed my parents' decision to ship him off to Uncle Harold and Aunt Helen's for several weeks. There is a photo of my brother and me posed in front of the Christmas tree years later. He is behind me, hoisting a toy rifle, a look of anger darkening his face. I look distracted as I push a baby doll stroller with large, black-gloved hands, my eyes cast to the side, my face solemn. His rage and my guilt, a division driven between us by circumstances over which we had no control.

I healed very quickly from the operation. Each night, my mother tucked me into a bassinet beside her bed, calling me her little dove. She said that she would wake up, and I'd be just lying there happily cooing. After those first few months home from the hospital, I was "no trouble," a delight—a good, quiet baby who could play for hours alone in my crib, pretending to read the books that she had given me.

And yes, I was very, very good. An intruder lived inside me though—the burden baby who might be dead.

In a haunting, recurring childhood nightmare, a brick dislodges from the edge of a hole in the foundation of a building, scattering thick dust that lingers ominously in the air. I'd wake up sweating, my heart racing, fearing that at any moment, the house would collapse.

By surviving the operation, I grew up believing that I had cheated death. By living, I was thumbing my nose at the Creator. God had wanted me to die, and I had disobeyed.

"Even though you had a stomach problem, I felt lucky to have a girl."

Even though.

"*You* birthed me," I remember blaming my mother when I was a teenager after she had criticized my dirty room.

"Yes, I did, didn't I?" she reflected, pausing in her vacuuming, holding the attachment perfectly still in the air between us, and tilting her head inquiringly as she contemplated this fact. She smiled mischievously, delighted with her discovery. "It certainly is my fault, yes. I can't deny it—I birthed you." We both laughed, but underneath my accusation, I was searching for the answer to an unasked question.

A milestone photo was taken of Dad and me when I made it to one year old—a close-up photo of our faces, his close to mine—a rare moment as he spent most of his time at home down the cellar in his workshop. He is a beaming full moon. Scrubbed and clean, he glows happily, his eyes smiling. I am happy, too, smiling what my mother calls a classic "buttermilk smile," no teeth but lips upturned. In front of us is a huge sheet cake, a mushroom candle at the center with a white shaft and a red cap with white polka dots. We celebrated. I had made it out of the danger zone.

One July 26th, my mother stepped out from the bathroom, blocking my way in the hallway, grabbed my upper arms and pulled me to her. Her hands gripped so tightly, I could feel each finger wrapped tightly around my bones. "You made it!" she declared.

I stood rock still, afraid to move.

"And I'm never going to let you go," she said, straightening her arms to hold me at arm's length and stare into my eyes, hers hard as marbles.

I froze, understanding the meaning of her words and actions: *You'll die if I let go.* Somehow, my life was still in danger.

There were tubes everywhere, in and out of every opening. —Mother

≈≈≈

My birthday was often celebrated down the shore as we vacationed there every July, staying with my Aunt Terry and Uncle Bill. It was a special time and place. Alone on top of the rocks across from their bungalow at Sandy Hook, New Jersey during childhood summers, with a view high up over the wide expanse of ocean, I felt most wholly myself. While other kids took swim lessons and played games on the beach, I hung out on the huge boulders that had been shipped in from Maine and piled up as a breakwater, each one weighing more than a ton. Blue sky unfurled as far as I could see, and at night, the brightly lit Coney Island Ferris wheel shimmered in the distance. The rocks were my furniture on my own outdoor porch: the special flat one on which I could lie comfortably on my side; the cupped one, like my father's armchair, on which I lounged; the one like a chair with a straight back where I sat and explored the vista with my father's clunky old binoculars. I loved searching the horizon for ships: tankers, luxury liners, fishing boats, and cargo ships. Sometimes I could actually read the name of a company painted on a ship's side.

Dashing across the tops of the rocks, I ran almost as fast as I could across land. One day, I found a secret cave where the water washed in from the crashing waves, a place I could see when I lay on my stomach and peered into a crevice. There, I waited for the ocean to bring me a treasure, a crab or a starfish; it never did. The cave was too high up and the water always washed everything back down to the sand. Yet I remained hopeful, thrilled by my own imaginings of what might appear.

On the rocks, the spray from the waves sometimes soaked me. I toasted in the sun, my skin turning gold, then reddening with freckles. I loved the contrast of my bronzed arm with the white sleeve of my T-shirt, loved by the sky, the salty wind, the waves that crashed wildly onto rocks, spray glinting silver in the sun, and the lacy white foam floating benignly on the swelling water once the wave receded. I was wild, basking in the aliveness that I could not bring into our bungalow, where it seemed that my mother wanted only the good me, the frozen one whom I thought of as dead.

At Sandy Hook, I got up early, the first human on the early morning wind-swept sand, where the footprints of gulls, three lines fanning out from a center point, were the only markings. The chill waves lapped rhythmically to shore. I walked barefoot along the shallow water where the gentle waves broke and the gulls' cries sliced the air. The bridge arched grandly in the distance. The town across the river was quiet.

Under my sweatshirt, I wore my stretchy, one-piece, black tank bathing suit with the three large, white buttons just beneath my breastbone. The sturdiness of the suit's material, a new type of synthetic, was comforting; it fit snugly and held me together in a way that made me feel safe. The buttons marking the place where the scar lived on my middle were my friends. It was as if the buttons and I had a pact; they would keep my secret. In my old cotton suit, the thin straps around my neck sometimes came undone in the surf. At any moment, I could be exposed. This new suit guaranteed that no one but the buttons and I knew that I was ugly underneath.

It was shady those early mornings, the sun hovering beyond the rock wall just above the ocean's horizon, and low tide at the river. I searched for something valuable among the necklaces of seaweed that traced the retreating arcs of high tide. Lots of small, clear blobs of jellyfish. Mussel shells, purple-edged. The stranded horseshoe crabs that I threw back into the sea. They could have actually walked back themselves but were slow, and I wanted to protect them from bathers at Sandlass' Beach Club who would soon cover the beach with colorful towels and umbrellas. People were cruel to the most vulnerable.

I love sea creatures. They look as if from some other time or place, especially those that come from way beneath the surface, shaped by the breath of water, wind, and waves, by currents and curtains of light, sand from the ocean's floor whipping up in all directions. Horseshoe crabs were plentiful on the river side of Sandy Hook. I watched them lumber slowly out of the sea and onto that peninsula jutting into the Atlantic Ocean. Unlike true crabs, they move forward, not sideways, and their horseshoe-shaped shells are much larger.

Horseshoe crabs, though fragile, are survivors. In the 450 million years Limulus Polyphemus, the scientific name, is known to have existed on this planet, this species has changed very little. Scientists often refer to them as "living fossils." Horseshoe crabs are not crustaceans but more closely related to arachnids, a group made up largely of spiders. They are hardy souls, like sponges, chitons—a mollusk whose shell is composed of eight plates—and coelacanths, an ancient fish that was thought to have gone extinct but that was discovered in the Indian Ocean in the '60s. I thought of them as miniature tanks plying the sand, yet easily crushed by a cruel boot. I have always identified with horseshoe crabs—vulnerable organisms, alien prehistoric-looking creatures that have persisted.

You looked like an alien from outer space! —Mother

Though they appear strange, horseshoe crabs have beautiful smooth, glistening, black shells, with two peaked ridges at the top, each housing a soft, black eye. A hinge at the back of the shell allows the lower part to flap, where a long, spiny, black tail attaches. Uncle Bill used to tell me to be careful when I was in the water because horseshoe crabs dig under the sand for camouflage, poking up their tails like spikes. "Do you want your foot to be like a marshmallow on a stick, little miss?" he'd laugh.

Uncle Bill's warnings intensified my fascination. Each morning I rushed my breakfast so I could race to the beach to see what the night tide had brought in. There they were, those slow ones, washed up at the high tide line. I picked up each one by its tail, a method I adopted to prevent its claws from grazing me, and gently flung it back into the water, careful not to dislodge the tail.

Once, I witnessed an older boy smashing a brick into a large, overturned crab. It lay on its back, helplessly flailing its legs and jabbing its tail into the sand as it attempted to right itself. Again and again the boy drew the brick back and hurled, crushing the guts and legs of the helpless creature. I wanted to stop the boy but was frozen, unable to move, somehow immobilized by what I was seeing. Later, I came upon the crab's wrecked body abandoned in the sand—its torn-up gut. I carried the crab to the water, set it right side up, and watched it sink into that element from which it came.

On the way back to the bungalow after those early morning walks, I passed a deep pit that my mother told me had been scooped out by a hurricane. Boulders, weathered boards, and pieces of fencing poked out of the sandy bowl. The ocean had lifted the boulders right off the rock wall across the street and plunked them down on the parked cars, my mother said—the same sea whose deep rhythmic *booms* lulled me nightly into sleep. That which crushed also soothed.

One summer, I found the small, white shell of a horseshoe crab on the beach under Fleischman's deck, where the sand is compacted and the color of Wheatena after it is cooked—black flecks amidst doe-brown grains. The shell was only eight inches long from the front edge to the tip of its tail; perhaps it was a baby and died young. A ghost, I thought, wondering if all baby horseshoe crabs were white or if what I had found was a molt, like a snake's. No traces were evident of the crab's body clinging to the shell.

Maybe the crab just slipped out.

As I picked it up, I felt uneasy about separating it from its impression in the sand. Its resting-place seemed sacred and inviolate, like a gravesite. I was strongly attracted to this crab, though. When I lifted it to the sun, it shone dully, capturing light, gathering and intensifying it, like a magnifying glass. I decided to keep the shell and stored it in a shoebox, looking in on it from time to time. *Did you die,* I wondered, *or did you merely leave your shell behind?* This question haunted me. *Dead or alive?*

I spent many hours exploring the coastline alone, walking barefoot in the shallow water along the river side of Sandy Hook. It was as though I was being pulled by an undertow. Some days, I was gone all afternoon. I wore my canvas Sandlass' Beach Club hat with the short brim, my white sweatshirt with the tiny-checked print on the front pouch and of course, my trusty black tank suit.

The sea was alive with its trillion blinking lights; the dark, clear, root beer–colored water; the tiny waves nipping at the shore; the shiny, buff-colored tube grass; the tufts of spiky dune grass; the clear blobs of jellyfish dotting the cool wet dark sand. I headed for the cove, that green water where the fat-bellied, yellow-green kellies swam, tracing the route I took with my father when we dragged for bait, and beyond. I was on a solo adventure, and my goal was reaching what I called the bomb shelter.

Along the beach, people sat on lawn chairs, usually in couples: a man and a woman beside one another, fishing poles stuck in rod holders in the sand nearby. The men resembled my father, short and wide-chested, wearing white T-shirts and caps with brims. But the women surprised me. Unlike my mother, they were stocky and short-haired, tough looking in their shorts and muscled legs. They talked tough, too. "How ya doin,' little gal?"

As I walked, I searched the beach and scanned the water for a bottle holding a note: *HELP, trapped on an island. Please come!* I was thinking of Popeye cartoons: X's floating on water marking the spot; Davy Jones's locker, a gray metal cabinet at the bottom of the sea; a bottle washing up with a note scrolled inside. Olive Oyl trapped on a very small island in the middle of nowhere with Popeye to the rescue. In every green Coke bottle, clear soda bottle, and brown beer bottle, I searched for a message. One time, I actually found a corked bottle with a paper inside. If there ever were any words, they had washed away, the square blank.

Once, I wrote my own note—crude, crooked letters to give the impression of physical weakness. I drew a rudimentary map, marking the four directions with arrows. I even pricked my finger with a sharp edge of tube grass and pressed the cut onto the page. Blood. I meant business. *HELP, HELP! PLEASE COME!* It was more than play.

Inevitably, I reached the "bomb shelter"—a small, abandoned brick building, the door long torn away, holes three feet wide perforating two walls opposite each other—perhaps a target test site for the Navy Base at the tip of the Hook? A strange buzzing sound sizzled in the air. Something compelled me to go in—some force that welled up from deep within—a need that had yet to be met. I stood for a moment as if frozen in time, then stepped up to the threshold. Could the shelter explode while I was inside? What lurked in those shadowy corners? What had made that oily spot on the floor? What could have happened here so many years ago?

Though frightened, I bolted in. A sinister-looking metal box hung on the shadowed wall, frayed wires dangling from its base. Was the place still juiced? Maybe a missile was heading for me right now! I could blow up, explode like a star, hunks of muscle and skin flying everywhere. I hunkered down, gritting my teeth, holding my breath, alert to a whistling sound. Time to get out! Don't be a sissy, I warned. It won't count if you leave too soon. You've got to be tough. You've got to feel as though you're as close to death as possible.

When I feared I'd break apart, I leaped out of the dark unscathed into the hot bright sand and punched my fists up into the air. I defeated the enemy! I had saved myself!

In a few days, though, I'd be back to do it all over again, an act over which I had no control. I was trying to heal myself, but I couldn't put the pieces together. How could I possibly know that I was reenacting an unresolved trauma? What drew me was beyond remembering. An unnameable power. I exploded once. Could I again?

At Sandy Hook, I was trying to heal myself with the help of the ocean, the river, and the creatures of the sea in an attempt to make myself whole again. Try as I might, though, I could not find relief or comfort for very long.

There were tubes everywhere, in and out of every opening. —Mother

Later, I would be drawn to sites of devastation. One Fourth of July, a group of friends and I saw an ambulance parked near a train overpass. A policeman told us that a boy had blown some of his fingers off, playing with fireworks. "Let that be a lesson t'ya," he warned. We scurried guiltily away, packs of firecrackers tucked into our waistbands and pockets.

For some reason, I felt compelled to find the site of the explosion and insisted that my boyfriend accompany me. Some boys pointed to the general vicinity where the accident occurred; amazingly, we found the exact place. Pieces of two fingers hung from the branch of a bush, blood coating the leaves. I quickly folded the chunks of skin inside a leaf, certain that they could be sewn back on, and rushed to the nearby fire station. The fireman told us that he'd put the remains on ice, promising to notify the police. "Perhaps something can be done," he said.

I knew my plan hadn't worked when in my first year of high school, the fingerless boy, Ozzie, became my square-dancing partner. When we circled, girls going one way and boys the other, the voice on the record called out, "Take that hand as you pass 'im by," and that was the hand I grabbed. We had both lost something important, our bodies irrevocably changed. His loss, though, was obvious and mine was a secret I bore.

One night before bedtime, reading my Nancy Drew book, I heard the waves pounding the rocks. The rain drummed the roof loudly, and I looked up nervously, hoping the roof was strong. A dark smudge dirtied the paint near the light fixture—a centipede with its pencil-thin body and a zillion legs sticking out the sides, one of the few insects that for some reason I was terrified of. The ceiling was low, the creature too close for comfort.

I stood on the bed on tiptoes and unscrewed the bolt holding up the glass cover. There it was—the brown gash. As I reached out to squash it with my tissue, it did the unthinkable: It dropped on me! I fell backwards onto the bed and over the side onto the throw rug.

I never did find that centipede. That night in bed with the light out, I squirmed, thinking it crawled on me under the covers. That night in a dream, the centipede crawled onto my abdomen right where my scar is and burrowed in, embedding itself like an anchovy on a pizza. Its tiny legs undulated, waving like kelp in underwater currents. I tried to pull it off, but for some reason, my hands couldn't reach my belly, and I woke up grabbing helplessly at the air.

Dusk along the river was magical—that in-between time of continual change, the sand cool on my feet. Just after dinner, we kids played running bases on the beach. It was thrilling to jump into the center, two playmates throwing the ball back and forth, closing in. Digging my sneakers into the cool sand, I pushed off for that sprint to home base. We played until the edges of the ball were no longer visible against the dimming light.

I stayed behind among the gathering shadows. I sat on the sand, hugging my knees, watching the lights in town wink on one by one across the Shrewsbury, burning bright and joyful against the darkening hills. The salty wind kicked up a chill. The small waves broke fast onto the shore, tide rushing in—*chew, chew, chew*. It was exciting to be so close to the unstoppable, relentless sea rising higher and higher. As the water blackened, I could never identify exactly when the lighthouse beacons lit up. Their dual towers lay white paths across the sea, coming straight to me as if I had been chosen. They activated this knowing inside me—that I was special and important simply because *I* existed.

These beams were solace when I was angry with my mother or father and I ran from the bungalow in tears, rushing to my familiar place in the sand, digging in my heels and staring intently into the light shimmering on the black water. I'll be a famous doctor when I grow up, I vowed, making lots of money, and when my parents come to me for help in their old age, I'll refuse. I was as hard as a giant clam then. I could not be pried open.

Nighttime in the bungalow, a kind of silky intimacy existed—a realm between life and death, a middle space between worlds. There were no doors on any of the first-floor rooms, only green curtains decorated with daisies. Between the kitchen and the living room was an open doorway, and no curtain hung across the opening to the staircase leading to the upstairs rooms where my mother, my father, Wayne, and I slept. There were no partitions upstairs either; in fact, next to my bed was a window that overlooked the staircase. It did have a shutter that could be opened and closed, but it never rested flush. This lack of privacy never seemed to be a problem. Down the shore, the infinite expanse of sky and water softened edges or did away with them altogether.

At dusk's end, as the day slid into night, my aunt, my mother, and I often sat on the porch in cane chairs that made a *crinch* sound when we shifted our bodies in them. How annoying. I was listening at a deeper level, like a shell at the bottom of the sea with my ear tuned to the currents. I heard the ocean's mighty heartbeat, a deep pounding that I felt inside my body. Outside the screens, lightning bugs reigned. People walked past on the sidewalk, laughing softly or talking in muted voices, thongs flip-flopping, sand crunching beneath shoes. We had a secret vantage point, the black screens acting like a one-way mirror; behind them, we were invisible to passersby.

On the wall behind us, dried starfish of a pale gold color were nailed onto the shingles. Some looked as if waving, others running. Several seemed to be leaping over hurdles. I imagined the starfish escaping, jumping off the wall and cartwheeling across the floor and down the steps. Turning like wheels, they rolled all the way down the sidewalk and over the sand to the Shrewsbury River, that place of brackish water where fresh water met salt, the home from which I imagined they had been plucked. As they entered the sea, they hissed a sigh of relief, a sound like when hot water meets cold. In that moment, they came back to life from the dead.

As a girl, I was drawn to whatever had been felled or broken apart as if some truth waited there to be revealed, knowledge that could rip open the shell of my life and rescue me from my dark shame. I would emerge innocent and pure, a free being of pearl.

A sunken ship lay at the bottom of the Shrewsbury. Locals said her masts were visible at low tide. Lore had it that it was a pirate vessel. Before the nation was born, pirates, Captain Kidd among them, hid in the coves of Sandy Hook and when a ship loaded with goods approached New York Harbor, they raced to plunder it. Toward the late afternoon at low tide, I squinted, hand shielding my eyes from the sun, searching for those spires. Mornings, I combed the beach for gold doubloons that, I'd heard, washed up on shore from time to time.

I had read about ghost ships that wandered the ocean, boats abandoned by crews, mere skeletons of vessels battered by wind and waves, emerging from time to time from the mists of the Bermuda Triangle, only to disappear again in the dusk-muted shadows. I knew about all types of sunken ships, from Roman galleys to the great sail ships.

When an older boy, Eddie, the son of the Petersons in the bungalow catty-corner to ours, pulled his speedboat onto the beach and asked if anyone wanted a ride, I practically dove into the boat. We sped to the middle of the Shrewsbury. What a thrill, the hull slapping the water and the spray soaking us. As he spun the boat around though, the motor suddenly died, and we floated at the mercy of the waves. "Damn rigging caught my propeller." So the story of the sunken ship was real! My stomach sank with fear. The dead boat was below, just out of sight, its ropes like eels looping around our legs. Could it take us down?

There were tubes everywhere, in and out of every opening. —Mother

He yanked and yanked on the engine's starter cord, but it was only when he had fiddled with the propeller and the boat drifted far enough away from the site that the motor caught.

The next day, I slipped under the ropes marking the swimming area and, powered by flippers, headed toward the sunken vessel. I was drawn to what was hidden, a story inside myself. Now that I realized it wasn't deep under the surface, I wore my mask, determined to see the ship's body. Perhaps I could even see a female figurehead, her life cut off at the waist. As I floated out beyond Fleishman's deck, the swells quickly carried me far from shore. The river was deep and the current strong, but it was something I felt compelled to do. As I neared the area where the ship went down, the sound of a motorboat, like a thirsty table saw, terrified me. If headed my way, they would never see me in time. Reluctantly, I turned back to shore. To this day, though, thoughts of that huge hulk belly-up at the bottom and the drowned maiden marking its bow stir me. What do they look like so many years after their fall? Is the ship mostly intact, the mast still upright? Or is it corroded, covered in seaweed and barnacles, sharks swimming in and out of its holes? Is the figurehead lying half-buried in sand? I was the sunken ship but didn't know it.

When I was twelve, the federal government reneged on a 99-year lease to the owner of Sandlass' Beach Club, and the Navy took possession of the Sandy Hook property. My uncle had the entire bungalow transported over the bridge across the Shrewsbury River on a trailer truck with my Uncle Bill, a telephone company lineman for Atlantic Bell, standing on its roof and shoving the telephone and electric wires away with a rod. They planted the house in a little town called Sea Witch, next to the Highlands, the larger town right across the river from the Hook where the house initially stood.

In the move, a part of me was locked into a suitcase and tossed overboard, left at the Hook—my world between life and death, where the river gave life and took life away and the booming ocean both threatened and soothed. There, on that thin spit of land, I had been closer to what I was inside—the part of me that felt alive and vital. In time, sand buried that case, and seaweed obscured the X marking the spot on the surface of the sea. A spirit secretly slept down there as if in a spell. Her breath rose and fell with the rhythm of the currents. She waited at the bottom of the sea to be brought back to life.

In Sea Witch, each night after dark, I surveyed the place where I'd been taken, walking moodily along the dock, kicking the gravel and sympathizing with the ships groaning in their moorings. I skulked along the bulkhead bordering the road at the end of our block, the crashing waves voicing my anguish. The sea was pure black, no lighthouse beams glittering on the water or lights shining from town across the river to cast sparkle onto the surface of the depths. We were in town.

There was something strange, almost haunted, about that place. Was the name Sea Witch from the days when Captain Kidd plied these waters and hid in the coves, Sea Witch the name of his sunken ship at the bottom of the Shrewsbury? Or maybe the town had simply been hexed. Many years earlier, my mother's father had secretly bought a bungalow in Sea Witch. He divorced my grandmother in the days when divorce was shameful and retreated there with his new wife. Soon after, he was found shot in the head, murdered by someone "in cahoots with his floozy," according to my mother. His death was recorded as a suicide, his money willed to his widow.

During the day, I sat on the beach, my eyes angry slits. The sand was fake, brought in by truck, and the small stream of sewage that ran perpendicular to the beach and into the surf smelled awful. I refused to swim there but instead, sat defiantly among the bathers, fully clothed, skipping pebbles across the water's surface. Late one afternoon when all the people were gone, I was surprised by a train of horseshoe crabs chugging along in the shallow water of the Shrewsbury, a large mother crab trailing her babies behind her. Each baby was attached to the one before it and ultimately, onto the skirt of the mother. For a moment I went soft, remembering those early days across the river of wonder and surprise. *Alive or dead?*

You looked like an alien from outer space! —Mother

My mother introduced me to a girl my age who lived next door, but I rejected her as plump, soft, dorky. I had become a tough kid by then, uncontrollable rage boiling up inside me. It was volcanic and steamed up from my origins. Angry words for my mother moved like glowing lava over the pages of my diary. Flames licked to life in my yard at home— fires I started by lighting heaps of pine needles and watching them burn. Where this anger came from, I did not know, but I wore a black leather jacket and roamed the streets at night, smoking cigarettes and drinking with friends on weekends.

That summer, I stole my father's switchblade from his dresser drawer and carried it in my pocket. The handle was buff-colored, made of bone, and curved slightly in an *S* shape. I kept my finger poised on the button that released the blade, alert to an ever-present danger. Give me a reason to cut you, my squinty, dark, cat-tailed eyes dared.

First Waters

We are one, after all, you and I, together we suffer, together exist, and forever will recreate each other. —Teilhard de Chardin

My mother's body is a battleground. I have listened to my mother's stories for decades, stories of great pain and sadness, stories of survival. As a child, I became lost in the intensity of her storm. In the force of her winds, it was hard to locate myself. My questions lifted into the sky like ocean spray and floated far away. Listening was my role.

At school, the teacher could rarely get me to speak. I nodded, shook my head. I was like a moon shell, the ocean roaring in my ears. In kindergarten, I sat by myself at snack time, just my milk and me. I focused on the red and white carton. The waxiness of its surface. How it was shaped like a little house. The pile of bubbles floating on the milk's surface. I was intent on sucking up the rich, white liquid through a straw and making sure I did not make a slurping noise when I got to the bottom. Every snack time was the same—the red carton and me.

Miss Anderson invited my mother in to speak with her. Why was I so shy, she wanted to know. After my mother told her about my operation, she had me sit with the same group of three children during snack and lunchtime. Slowly, I began to play with others in the playhouse and in the sandbox. I wouldn't push my toy truck in the circle with the other children while the sounds of honking horns played on the phonograph, but I did begin to assert myself. When Miss Anderson asked who wanted to play the sandpaper blocks with the "orchestra" during music time, I raised my hand.

The story of a woman's body cannot be told without telling the story of her mother's. The seed of my relationship with my body was planted by my mother. Anyone who ever met her knows about the abuse she suffered at the hands of her father. My mother's body is a beaten one. Her bruising started at a young age. I have heard her tell total strangers as we sat in a doctor's office or waited in a grocery line about her father smacking her face until her nose bled, about him stropping her bare legs until they bled. It was as early as age three or four that I remember hearing my mother's tales. As she washed clothes in the cellar, a time-consuming act in the fifties, and I played nearby with my dolls, I heard the stories of my mother's pain. It was as if she was talking to herself and I overheard. On automatic, she uttered phrases that she has used time in and time out. These same phrases offer themselves to me now when I am fifty and my mother ninety.

Just the other day, she berated herself: "I could just hit myself. I could just take a paddle and whack myself. I just want to hit myself everywhere, I am so angry. How could I be so stupid?"

"Mom, you're ninety. Give yourself a break," I pleaded.

"Not until I'm in my grave."

As a twelve-year-old, she spent most summer afternoons at the German Turnverein, a gymnastics club in Newark, New Jersey. She took a bad fall from the parallel bars one day onto her neck and walked the mile home from the gym "bent over like the Hunchback of Notre Dame." Her mother scolded her for hurting herself and sent her to her room.

One fall morning during that same year, she watched her father pull a pistol from a drawer and place the tip of the barrel against her mother's temple. "Go to school," he ordered as she backed out the door, intent on keeping her mother in sight for as long as she could. All the way up the block, she listened for gunshots. At school, she heard nothing the teacher said. When the bell sounded, she ran home and upon seeing her mother in the front yard, sank down on the sidewalk, overcome with relief. Nothing was ever said about the incident.

I was filled with hatred for this man at a very early age. I still do not know how to forgive him or whether I want to. I come close when I think of him as a child hanging by his thumbs from the kitchen trapdoor into the dark, damp root cellar—his father's punishment of him for infractions.

There is no tombstone on his grave. For many years, I have wanted to put one there, not out of respect or love, but simply to do what one ought to for the dead. But when I bring up the subject, my mother always says, "This is what we agreed to, my brothers and I. This is what we want."

She learned early on that she had to rely on herself. There was no one to help. She won an essay contest for a piece she wrote about her dog Jack. "Five dollars was a lot in those days," she told me proudly. The day she was awarded the certificate and prize money from Haynes and Company at a special ceremony at the store, not one of her family members accompanied her.

Alone, she checked into a hospital in her early twenties for surgery that would remove a tumor on her ovary. She agreed to an experimental anesthetic because ether made her very ill. Initially when she awoke from surgery, she was deaf, having suffered nerve damage. Gradually she regained her ability to hear, but the racket never went away and drowned out much of her hearing. Hearing aids helped.

After reading Poe's poem "The Bells" in the seventh grade, I thought of my mother's condition as "tintinnabulation." Certainly, Poe had not meant the kinds of bells my mother heard in her ears, the clang of tinnitus. "I wish you could hear them, Wend," she said, "a real cacophony. Loud bells, soft bells, fast bells, slow bells—I've got everything."

"I am beside myself," I have often heard her say; she has never moved into her body. Hours before minor surgery on her nose, she looked in the mirror, saying, "I have always hated this schnoz. I hope they take it off."

It is as if my mother is not aware that she has a body until she has injured it. I have often seen her reach for something only to crash her hip, knee, or elbow into a table or shelf simply because she didn't take into account the fact that an object might be in between her and the thing she wanted. Caring for her body is low priority. Rubbing lotion on her hands and elbows after washing the dishes or lying down for a half hour at the end of the day to rest her aching back is my mother's idea of pampering. She goes to the doctor when the pain is so bad she can't walk or move her arm or chew food or lift her head. Bodies are burdens. Bodies are inconvenient. Bodies are to be conquered.

When my mother talked about her pregnancies, it was as if she was a World War II veteran who had returned from the bloodiest battlefields. Her tone was somber as she narrated the details of each tragedy. Six months into her first pregnancy, she miscarried during a hurricane in Florida. My mother called this her "blue baby incident" and claimed Roger would have lived had an incubator been available. At the time, she was living with my father on the naval base, later renamed Cape Canaveral, and was hospitalized after contracting a high fever. According to my mother, the doctors never treated her, just fed her navy beans as she lay suffering. Hours before the storm, patients thought to be the most seriously ill were flown out; then the base's airplanes were moved to safety, so there was no way to transport my mother from the naval hospital to a place where a premature infant could be properly cared for.

After she lost the baby, my mother, furious at the Navy and the hospital, demanded that they discharge her in the middle of the hurricane and that my father take her home. He convinced his commander to let him drive her from the naval facility. The car blew all over the road as large metal barrels flew past their windows. She didn't really care about living at that point, she told me. Back at their apartment, the windows banged, threatening to blow off their hinges, and water poured through the roof. There was nothing to eat except leftover hamburger that my father broke into pieces and hand-fed her. I liked knowing this about my father and hearing the tenderness in my mother's voice as she told this part of the story. I loved my father for helping her in this way.

When the Navy insisted that my father pay for burial of the baby, he confronted his commanding officer, a pistol concealed beneath his coat. He never had to use the gun. The commander liked my father and convinced the higher-ups to sign a paper authorizing the Navy to pay.

During the second pregnancy, my mother's labor pains began when she and my father were vacationing in Sandy Hook and a storm was coming in. Medical facilities were far away, so my mother and father left, thinking they could get ahead of the deluge. In the intense rain, a car sideswiped them. My mother said that the car was ripped in half literally from front to back and that they landed three lanes over facing the opposite direction. Luckily, no cars were coming.

However, as the car spun, and Red Dog, their seventy-pound Irish setter, was thrown violently against her, my mother's placenta was damaged. Why the doctor beat on her belly to abort the baby I don't know, but according to my mother, he injured her bladder. The baby lived almost four hours in the incubator, then died. For years after the accident, she suffered attacks of toxic poisoning, paralyzing a different part of her body with each attack, a condition resulting from not being cleaned out properly after the doctor had aborted her placenta. Poison had entered her bloodstream. She bore the condition for years, unwilling to seek help from doctors. They were the ones who she felt caused the problem in the first place, and she would not subject herself to more "torture."

My parents gave up trying to have children. When my mother became pregnant with Wayne ten years later, she was shocked. After three months of pregnancy, the doctor ordered her to lie down as much as she could so that she could bring the baby to full term. Apparently due to some glitch with her body, whether physical or hormonal, if she weren't careful, the baby could slip out prematurely. When mom's water broke, she couldn't keep Wayne from being born in the back seat of their car as my father rushed to the hospital. He had ingested radiator fluid that had pooled on the seat from car parts my father had stored there. Wayne spent his first days in an incubator. No one knew whether he'd pull through.

I was the least tragic birth. My mother had just gotten to the hospital and upstairs when I was born, my father still standing at the nurses' station signing the papers. When he got the news that he had a baby girl, his knees gave out. He grabbed the counter before he went down. The shock of how fast I'd come took over.

When I was small, I played in the basement in the dimness of two light bulbs as my mother did the laundry nearby. I heard her talk to herself about the deaths of her first two babies. Maybe the cave-like, more primitive surroundings opened the old wound. She wept, dabbing her eyes with tissues, as she delivered the stories of her losses. After a few loads, the floor was littered with crumpled Kleenex, a scattering of white roses. Witnessing her grief convinced me that these babies were the ones that she had wanted, not Wayne and me.

I would have no babies, I decided at a very young age. Birth was a battleground where the dead lay rotting, and the wounded struggled to survive. No one walked away unscathed if one walked away at all.

My mother had a different sense of herself when she talked about Greenwood Lake, a large body of water shared by northern New Jersey and southern New York State where her father owned property and where she experienced the happiest times of her life—a rare wholeness radiated from her body when she spoke of it. She loved to be alone in nature. As a teen, she took a basket and her forked stick as a protection against snakes and hiked the trails around the lake and up into the surrounding mountains alone, listening for the sounds of boats' motors to find her direction. She gathered wildflowers, roots and all, and at the end of the day, replanted them around the small bungalow her family owned. Her favorite place was a huge rock atop the opposite mountain. It took all day to hike there and back, and often my mother was late for dinner. The family didn't even notice that she was gone. "You must remember," she said flatly, "there were six of us." Nature was a loving parent for my mother.

When I was a little girl, my mother invited me into her relationship with the outdoors—her tulips lining the front walk; the mountain ash that she planted with its orange berries; the garden with its leafy lettuces and large red tomatoes. I weeded and watered. She taught me to aim the spray at the base of the plant and not at the blossom. While my mother knelt, digging her trowel into the dark, rich soil, I raked up the pine needles and horse chestnut leaves, pulled dandelions, and clipped grass to make a neat edge along the silver, glittery rocks we had gathered from the shore to decorate the garden.

Our play, though, was parallel—she on her side of the yard and me on mine. When I tried to kneel next to her as she picked tomatoes, she shooed me off. "Water the roses for me, will you Wend?" I wanted to be near her, doing things side by side, both of us knees down in dirt, but she would not have it. "Here, hon, take this hose and water the geraniums in the pot near the porch." I complied. I was a good girl, but I longed to cross over into my mother's world—a world I sensed was there. Sadly, entry was blocked, so separate we remained.

I have never been to Greenwood Lake. My mother never took my brother or me hiking in any woods to share her love of the forest and the mountains. When I was five years old, I overheard my mother talking to my father about Greenwood Lake while riding in the back seat of the old Ford. Brimming with excitement, I sprang forward, my hands grasping the back of my mother's seat: "Can we go there for vacation, to the mountains?"

After a long pause, my mother said cautiously, "We'll see." This meant no, and I knew that an explanation would never be given.

The wall between my mother and me crumbled briefly when I was three years old. At the ocean, my mother, as usual, was sitting on her beach chair reading a thick, plastic-covered book from the library while I played alone in the sand with my pails and shovels and Wayne rode the waves in the surf. I was digging my shovel into the wet sand, trying to capture a sand crab, but again and again the shovel came up empty. My mother must have seen my frustration because suddenly, she was kneeling beside me, her hand rigid like a trowel. She jammed her fingers quickly and deeply into the wet sand, tunneling straight down, and then yanked up. There in her palm was a sand crab! She dropped it into my hand.

This crab was so different from the usual type in which legs radiate out from a flat shell. This crab was gray and tubular, tapered like a bullet, with lots of tiny legs bunched together at the end opposite the tip, like a squid, and much larger than I would have thought given the size of the hole. Together we marveled at the strangeness of the tiny creature momentarily in our grasp.

"Time to set it free," my mother urged. I balked, not wanting to relinquish this shared intimacy. "Let it go." Impatience edged her voice. Reluctantly, I opened my hand. Even now I feel regret, for I never was able to capture another. Would I have been satisfied even if I had? It was my mother's presence next to me in shared communion that I wanted.

∽∽∽

Every Thanksgiving, my mother and I made pies together. As I stood on the stepstool flattening dough onto a cutting board with a rolling pin, she showed me how to slide the flipper carefully under the pale circle, lift it just so and drape it over the glass pie dish. I liked pressing the dough gently into the dish and folding it over the lip. But as soon as she began crimping the edges of the piecrust, I felt dread.

"After the operation," she'd explain, "the surgeon met with me in his office and showed me exactly what he'd done." She picked up a yellow #2 and clasped it lightly in a horizontal position between her thumb and index finger, the other three fingers extended with poise. "He held out a pencil like this." Pointing to the pencil tip for emphasis, as the surgeon had probably done, she said, "The opening of the valve was no bigger than that of a pencil lead and had to be widened." She pinched the air near the pencil tip and pretended to unfold something, then pinched and unfolded again, mimicking the surgeon peeling back the thick muscle. "Like folding the dough over when making a pie crust," she said. Then she pretend-stitched the skin into place around the outside of the pencil as the surgeon did around the outside of the valve.

The operation was "delicate," my mother said he had told her, the instruments very tiny. "You had stitches on the outside and stitches on the inside," Mom said, "which is why it was so crucial that you not cry and break them. Day and night we watched over you, picking you up over the slightest little thing." She then placed the pencil carefully onto the table, holding it for a moment with her fingertips, her face serious, her eyes looking away, focused on scenes from an inner movie. She was reliving something, settling unfinished business. Was she weighing the sacrifices? Slowly she lifted her hand. The spell was broken. There we were—she and I poised over the partially crimped crust.

The scar from my early surgery symbolized our relationship—flawed, interrupted. The only time my mother mentioned it was to complain about its size. I might be toweling off after a bath or dressing after a swim at Linden Pool when she'd remark: "Gee, Wend, it's too bad that scar keeps on stretching."

As a girl, I fantasized ways to make it disappear: applying makeup to it; erasing it like a pencil mark; or massaging it into my skin as if my stomach were made of Play Dough. Maybe one day, it would straighten its legs and hop away, like a grasshopper. Other scars on my body eventually vanished, I told myself, or left only the slightest trace. This scar, though, was here to stay. A spider's spinnings, crazy webs on my belly that lengthened and widened over time. My scar seemed a raggedy job—octopus legs fused onto my skin. A tendril of red algae ripped from its holdfast. I was stamped— DAMAGED GOODS.

My mother modeled perfectionism. During the school year, I was her dress-up doll, hair pulled neatly into a ponytail, spiraling into one long baloney curl. Or she prodded the one curl into many, lying neatly on my shoulders. She packaged me in cute dresses: the gray one with the "bolero collar" or the "eggshell" white dress with the black piping and yellow flowers. Matching socks and shiny patent leather shoes completed the outfit. "My little doll," she called me.

At school, I was a little lady: legs crossed, arms pressed close to my body, silent unless spoken to. I earned A's in reading, spelling, handwriting, arithmetic, drama, gym, and art. The teachers' comments on the backs of my report cards read: "a delight," "a dream," "a pleasure." The pressure from within and without to maintain this role was relentless.

Sometimes the pressure was relaxed, and my mother gave in to my being a child. Before I said my prayers, she let me jump up and down on my bed. It was a special time for us. Standing beside me while I jumped, she pressed my shoulders down just as my feet touched the mattress, popping me up like a Jack in the Box. On the next bounce, she pushed again, harder. Once I got a good rhythm going, she pushed down on the bed each time my feet hit the mattress, intensifying each bounce. My mother and I were in synch, abandoned to the physics of motion. She shook her head. "The springs, Wend," she worried, "the springs!" I shrugged. She rolled her eyes and laughed. She kept pushing.

Perfection, I decided, would absolve me, make up for the pain I had caused. A little girl died then and another was born. Requiring nothing of anyone, I would be the most wonderful little girl around. Mother's best helper.

While my mother food shopped, I transformed the house. In the living room, I polished the fireplace brass; dusted every item and surface; vacuumed the carpet; shook out the throw rugs; straightened the paintings on the wall; and beat the pillows and cushions in the fresh air to make them plump and dust-free. I swept the kitchen floor, dusted the shelves in the bathroom, and refolded the towels. As soon as my mother arrived home, I raced out to the car to help with the packages. As I put them down on the kitchen table, I heard her exclaim as she walked through the house: "How beautiful! How hard you worked. Look at this bathroom!" I was a good girl. I had been worth saving.

Inside, I felt confused. I was a sickly little girl/I was a perfect little girl. An ugly baby/a good baby. A burden baby/a dream baby. A plug nickel girl/a miracle girl. A problem/a delight. The sand kept shifting. I could not find a solid place to plant my feet.

Like my mother, I have been at war with my body for as long as I can remember. My body betrayed me early on, so I ran away. There have been truces, periods of tolerance, some forgiveness lately, but overall, a steady siege of repulsion and rage has rained down.

Early in life, I was obsessed with splitting my skin. As a young girl, I used teeth and fingernails. Ruthlessly, I bit off ragged cuticles with my front teeth and tore skin off my feet after bathing while my heels and toes were soft. I dug out scabs and pimples until they bled. Chunks of cheek bitten away from inside my mouth caused my dentist consternation. During one exam, he called my mother into the room. "Open wide," he said, pressing my tongue down with a wooden stick. He reached his thumb into my mouth and folded my cheek back so that the inner wall showed. My mother's lower jaw dropped—"Looks like the Grand Canyon." "She's ripped up the other side as well," he said grimly.

When I was five, I treasured a penknife with a multi-colored handle that my father had given me. I called it my Lifesaver knife because it reminded me of the variety of colors in the packet of Lifesaver suckers called "mixed fruit." When a neighbor boy, who terrorized me every chance he got, tore the head off my baby doll, I stabbed at his hand as he leaned on our picnic table, his fingers splayed. He pulled away just in time, the blade jabbing into wood instead. "She tried to kill me!" he yelled, pointing at me. "She tried to stab me with a knife!" I burned with shame at his public outcry. I too was shocked at what I'd done; it just seemed to happen. What really surprised me though was the delight that I had felt as I lashed out. I tucked this knife into the vanity table drawer, afraid of the harm I might cause.

Juggling knives became a compulsion—a habit that satisfied some unknown need. When I was eleven and just home from school, my mother and father still at work, I'd pull out the knife drawer and choose my weapons: the cleaver or "butcher knife" as Mom called it, a rectangular-shaped blade used for chopping, and the steak knife, the mean-looking one with the razor-like blade that Dad sharpened regularly on the grinding wheel. Just like I'd seen at Asbury Park, an amusement park down the shore, I began with the master of ceremonies' words: "Ladies and Gentlemen and children of all ages, step right up and see the death-defying feats of the knife juggler!" I mastered flipping the steak knife one full circle in the air and catching it by the handle. I could even do it at different speeds. The finale was a super slow-motion flip three feet over my head and the catch—just before it hit the floor.

Juggling two knives was harder. I practiced passing one knife from my left hand to my right so the transfer, while the other one was in the air, would be second nature. Then, a knife in each hand, I'd flip up the one in my right hand, switch the other from left to right, and catch the descending knife with my left. This I could do, but I could not manage two knives in the air at once. As one descended and the other rose, I lost my concentration. Catching one, the other clattered to the floor. Once I stuck out my knee to break its fall—my mother would kill me if I cracked the handle or worse, scarred the linoleum. The tip plummeted into my thigh and fell woodenly to the side; oddly, my skin was not cut.

My best feat was to balance the cleaver on my nose. I set the tip of the blade on the bridge and leaned my head back, dancing to keep the knife upright, lunging back and forth, bent-kneed, a slave to gravity's pull. Then, I snapped my head upward, which pitched the cleaver into the air as I stepped back. I grabbed the falling handle with a flourish and bowed deeply, brandishing the cleaver. See? Knives can't hurt me! I've got them under my control. I wonder now, whom was I performing for? Later in life, I realized my obsession with knives was my attempt to take back my power. As a baby, I was helpless under the surgeon's scalpel. As I grew up, if anyone would be doing the cutting, it would be me.

I still pick ruthlessly at myself, tearing at cuticles, scraping the soles of my feet with my fingernails, digging into my ears and nostrils, ripping off old blisters, biting off pieces of skin from my lips. I just can't seem to leave myself alone. What if I stopped biting, picking, ripping, tearing, poking, peeling, scraping, gouging? What if I stopped hurting myself? A world would die. A world would be born.

∼∼∼

Recently, I read the book *Hannah's Gift,* about the life of a young child with cancer and the changes her family went through. At one point, three-year-old Hannah is having a birthday party soon after coming home from the hospital, where a tumor had been removed from her abdomen. The staples were still holding her incision closed. When her small friends gathered in the house after a treasure hunt in the yard, the atmosphere was tense. No one brought up the subject of Hannah's illness. But Hannah broke the ice simply by lifting up her dress and saying, "'Hey, you guys, do you want to see my scar?'" The little girls bubbled with questions. Hannah answered them honestly, with authority and humor. One girl was even jealous. "'Wow, I want to have surgery!'" she said. When the hubbub died down, Hannah gracefully lowered her dress, and the party continued.

The summer of my thirteenth year, two-piece bathing suits were in, one-piece bathing suits simply not for sale in most stores. There was no foolproof way to hide my scar. "What is that?" my friends asked, pointing at my middle. My voice went on automatic monotone. *When I was twenty-six days old, I had pyloric stenosis. My stomach valve was closed between the stomach and small intestine, and I wasn't digesting my food, so they had to operate.* This reportage ended the discussion. I was a closed book; don't dare try to open it.

In my life, scars meant imperfection. Scars weighed my family down with burdens it couldn't carry.

As a teenager, exhausted by my obsession with perfection, I tried disruption. Troubled, I reached for trouble. I latched onto the black leather jacket crowd—a quick descent to hell.

When I first slipped a razor blade out of its cardboard cover, admiring its shiny edge, and sliced the curve of the letter "G" into my forearm, the first initial of my boyfriend's name, I didn't want to cut too deeply; this would hurt. Cutting lightly with a razor only stung. Once, I cut his whole first name in capital letters. I concentrated deeply, slicing just enough to feel a slight burn. Feeling a little pain was better than feeling nothing at all. *Alive, not dead.*

I also carved "CS," my best friend's initials. Blood beaded along the cuts and sometimes spilled over. When finished, the skin around the initials was puffy and vulnerable. I felt sorry for myself then and could nurse my wounds. To prevent infection, I poured on alcohol that stung sharply. Then, I rubbed on soothing antibiotic ointment and draped Band-Aids over the incisions. I felt comforted and cared for.

I only wanted to slash my wrist a little. I was drinking with the gang, my new friends, partying at my house before school one morning. My mother had left for work at seven and by eight o'clock, the living room was crowded with kids and smoke. By nine a.m., I was pretty drunk and couldn't control the razor. I gouged at my veins, splitting skin, amazed at how quickly it peeled away from the cut, like paper on fire. A wide, red opening gaped, shocking me. Blood poured into the sink.

The party came to an abrupt halt, Bobby ushering everyone out the front door. My friend Karen stayed behind to help. We took a taxi to the emergency room, where I told the nurse that I cut my wrist slicing bread. I modeled holding up the loaf of rye just so, the slipping of the blade. She secured the wound with butterfly Band-Aids and wrapped my wrist with gauze. "Keep it clean," she warned. I do not know what she wrote in her report, but my parents never mentioned it. They did not seem to notice the white bandage that I hid under the length of my shirtsleeve.

That night, I hung out with some of the gang at the pizza parlor and afterward, walked home alone in a light drizzle, aware of my extreme vulnerability—how easily the cut could split open. I paused for a moment on Baker Street, remembering my friend telling me about his father chasing him with a knife down this very sidewalk. Life was precarious. The rain seemed to sympathize. I have always felt understood by rain.

That summer, I told my mother that I was staying down the shore in Lavallette with my friend Michelle and her mother. Michelle and I bummed a ride down the Parkway with some kids in a stolen car. I got so drunk along the way that I hung my head out the window as we drove over the bridge into Matawan and threw up onto the side of the car.

During the day, we begged for spare change on the boardwalk and at night, slept at Pat's place. Pat owned an apartment building and a Laundromat. He let Ann, a young girl who had run away from home and who was trying to make it by working as a waitress, stay in one of his apartments for free, and she, in turn, let us girls stay with her.

Later we figured out that Pat was a pimp. We were hanging out at Pat's place when "his girls" came back to his apartment at two a.m. after working the boardwalk. They threw some cash down on the kitchen table and flopped onto the sofa, lighting up cigs. "What are you girls doin' here?" one asked. "Pat, you pimpin' kids now?" We put two and two together.

We ate breakfast each morning at the corner store: Yodels, prepackaged apple turnovers, and coffee. Dinners were pork roll on a bun with mustard that we bought near the Wild Mouse, a ride where the cars tilted out over the ocean at the end of the pier. Every so often, the riders' screams could be heard over the bells and buzzers of the boardwalk games.

Pat's place was about a half mile from the boardwalk, so we hitched rides. One guy who picked Mary and me up pulled out his dick shortly after we got in the car and played with himself while driving. I elbowed Michelle who was sitting next to the car door and nodded toward his dick. We had strategies for these types of encounters. At the stoplight, she quietly pushed down on the door handle and at her cue, we rolled out into the street. Another time, running from a pack of drunken boys, we jumped into the back of a teal blue pickup that stopped for us. Sometimes, I ended up drunk at parties, not knowing how I got there or how I would ever get back to Pat's.

One morning, Michelle and I found ourselves with two guys in a parking lot, sitting in the open back of a VW van turned psychedelic bus. "Coming to me in the Morning," a song by Cream, blasted from the bus's speakers. Michelle and I had met them at Flo's All Night Diner. We had taken mescaline with them on the beach at about two a.m. and had watched the sunrise, smeary yellow and orange.

My hair was tangled, my body unwashed, my teeth unbrushed, my mouth sour from chain-smoking. I felt honest, raw, and real. I was on the outside what I felt like inside. Since the water had stopped running in Ann's apartment, we took a bar of soap to the ocean once a week. Washing in salt water does not make you feel clean.

Michelle and I caught a ride back to Hillside, our hometown, with a friend of Pat's, a man who drank whiskey all the way up the New Jersey Parkway while driving in a torrential storm. He had one of those cars with a speedometer built into the steering column that looked like a 3-D map of space. Each 10-mph jump in speed was a separate illuminated orbit. The car's speed lit up in red numbers. The warm yellow light within the chamber calmed me. I stared at this dashboard drama all the way up the Parkway to keep me from thinking about the car wreck we were headed for. The rhythm of the windshield wipers beating back and forth soothed me. When he pulled off Route 22 and into Super Diner's parking lot, I was amazed. We were alive and had made it back to Hillside. The rain had stopped and I was about a mile away from home. As soon as I walked in the door, my mother grounded me. While Michelle and I were away, she had bumped into Michelle's mother food shopping at the Acme Market. It was a case of 2 + 2.

That winter, my friend J.P. was killed, his head severed from his body as he played chicken near the overpass on Route 22. In the spring, Jerry, my best friend Cheryl's boyfriend, committed suicide, swallowing mercury he took from the thermometer of his parents' washing machine. My friend Jimmy got shipped off to the Marlboro, a kind of penitentiary for teen boys. Another friend, Margie, got pregnant and sent to a convent. I got kicked out of school for playing hooky, so my mother grounded me from seeing my boyfriend and hanging out with my friends. In a meeting with the school psychologist, he told me that my mother was considering sending me away to a convent.

One drizzly afternoon while my parents were at work and I was home ironing clothes, one of my weekly chores, and watching *Concentration*, the TV game show, I swallowed thirty aspirin. The weird feeling of nausea and bloating was more than I bargained for—bubbles grew in my gut but never popped. Bubbles and more bubbles. I had just turned fourteen. I was ready to try perfect girl again.

The Intertidal Zone

When we go down to the low-tide line, we enter a world that is as old as the earth itself—the primeval meeting place of the elements of earth and water, a place of compromise and conflict and eternal change. —Rachel Carson

At age sixteen, I became an environmentalist. *Oceans Magazine* had delivered news that I could not ignore. In Louisiana, scientists discovered that pelican eggs were cracking long before the progeny hatched. Paper thin, the shells could not hold. DDT was the culprit as Rachel Carson had warned in *Silent Spring*. It was 1969. I presented my report about the pelicans to my high school honors biology class, showing photos of mother birds standing over cracked eggs—pelicans dead before they were born. Dead babies. Dead babies everywhere.

I would major in biology and save the pelicans. I would fix that which was broken; help those hurt before their lives had even begun; prevent the pain of future generations. I subscribed to *Ocean's Magazine*, watched Jacques Cousteau and nature films on TV, and tacked photos of scuba divers onto the bulletin board over my desk. I applied to schools that boasted superior programs. The University of Miami accepted me.

No matter that U of M was considered a party school by north-easterners and that many of my friends were headed for Ivy League schools. No matter that both my best friend and the boy I was in love with were staying home to attend local colleges. I was heading off on a 747 into the blue unknown, leaving my old life behind. Lured by field stations in the Keys and South

America, the international reputation of the graduate school, the research vessel, and the distance from home, I booked my flight.

Science promised stability. On exams, blank lines awaited correct answers: the scientific name of a carbon polymer; the acronym that stood for the double helix; the term for algae and fungi living in symbiosis. Every question was answerable, every mystery solvable. I wanted that perfect clarity: things were alive or dead, right or wrong, open or closed.

A deeper question drove me though, a question of which I had no conscious knowledge—why was I born broken?

Freshman year at the University of Miami was a crazy time—an intertidal zone of ocean, where sea life and debris were tossed and shaken by the pounding surf, subjected to great turbulence. I could not get my footing, a situation that was becoming a repeating theme in my life. I had no idea that I held a life-threatening belief about myself—that I was broken and incapable of becoming whole. I did not know how strongly I attracted other broken beings and that these types of liaisons largely controlled my life. I was subject to rip tides and strong currents that others seemed to miraculously bypass.

One of my biology professors, Dr. Jergens, described several theories about the origin of living beings. Perhaps life plummeted to earth on a meteor, the rock acting as a tiny spaceship, transporting the genetic material, maybe in the form of primitive bacteria. Maybe chemicals in the water, originating from the volcanic spewing of early earth, formed compounds that were one day zapped by lightning and an amino acid was formed. Thus, life began as a primitive aggregate floating in the water. This idea was a particular favorite as a scientist at the University of Miami's graduate school had conducted many of the experiments that corroborated these findings. When Dr. J. lectured on the origins of life, he gave it a mystical bent, which intrigued me. He urged us to read Teilhard de Chardin, a paleontologist who wrote about the evolution of the spirit. I bought the pale, blue paperback *The Phenomenon of Man* but was unsuccessful at penetrating its meaning. Nevertheless, I knew that at the end of the day, when you boiled it all down, life—all life—seemed to come from the sea.

But how exactly had human beings evolved from this first aggregate floating on top of a vast ocean? How did we become bipeds, strolling along the beach at dusk? And why do some species thrive and others struggle?

Socially, I was lost at the U of M. Trying to fit in and do what girls did on a Friday night, I went to a frat party where, I discovered, drunken, blonde, well-built boys were out on the make for drunken, blonde, skinny girls. Where did I fit in with my auburn hair and plump thighs? At one point, I was herded into a smoky room where boys lined up along one wall. Apparently, we girls were supposed to make out with them, assembly-line fashion. I left.

I walked the blocks around fraternity row in tears, the light of the full moon illuminating the cumulus clouds floating close to earth, much closer than I'd ever seen in New Jersey. The palms cut dramatic silhouettes into the huge bright clouds. How odd these trees were to me then. Where were the oaks and maples of my youth? Why was I so far away?

In my personal version of the *Scala Naturae*, a chart that Aristotle created to show a hierarchical relationship between all creatures on the earth with man lording over all, I put the human mind at the top and the human body at the very bottom, along with the bacteria. Bodies malfunction. Bodies betray. Bodies are reminders of pain. I hung large shirts over mine and only paid attention to it when I was hungry or under extreme circumstances, like when I had to walk through a knee-high flood of water to get to class. I acknowledged my body only when I could not manage to ignore it.

After a month of eating all I wanted each meal at the student dining room and gaining fifteen pounds, I resorted to the Atkins Diet: eggs, meat, ketchup, and salad. As a result, toxic nitrogenous byproducts built up, necessitating a continual flushing of the system: water, water, and more water. I chain-smoked and lived on coffee, doctored with a huge heap of Coffee Mate and refined white sugar. I felt bloated and spacey, but I looked great. Boys noticed me.

One called nightly, serenading me by imitating Mick Jagger. Why I dutifully listened, I don't know. Sometimes I set the receiver onto the counter for a whole five minutes while I went to the bathroom or talked to someone in the hallway, yet when I picked it back up, he was still yelling hoarsely.

Another, Jacob, sought a platonic friendship: he never made a pass at me or even sent the slightest sexual innuendo in my direction. We shared dinner each night in Pearson Hall, complaining about the heavy course load in the CORE science major program and reporting on the rumored sexploits of others, notably the nightly drama of tiny Suzie with three hundred pound Mitchell—his fucking her up against the wall of his shower.

Jacob and I had one off-campus date. I agreed to accompany him to a big frat party that he was desperate to go to. As he could not hold his liquor and passed out on the deck of the swimming pool, I ended up walking back to the dorm drunk and alone along the railroad tracks bordering Ponce de Leon Boulevard. Shortly after, he changed his major from bio to business, and we lost touch.

Lenny Lee from Hong Kong was my most steady male partner, though he too sought no sexual favor that I could discern. Nightly at eleven p.m. sharp, Lenny secured a box to his bike rack and we headed off campus on our bicycles, hunting mangoes from the backyards of the surrounding neighborhoods. He climbed the fences, plucked the fruits, and tossed them to me for packing. I felt bad stealing from innocent sleepers and from time to time worried that we were going to get caught. "What can they possibly do to us?" Lenny insisted. "This is America. Jail university students for stealing fruit?"

"Stealing is stealing," I countered. I don't think Lenny believed that anyone from his background—private schools in London, his father a physician—could be penalized for a trivial misdemeanor. "What makes you above the law?" To this, he shrugged his shoulders, but for some reason, I continued to accompany him. The warm, moonlit jasmine-scented nights. The thrill of getting away from campus. The challenge of flying down the slate sidewalk along Douglas Boulevard, ducking the slaps of overarching palm branches. Lenny and I were buddies, two kids far from home.

∽∽∽

"Catfish are cousins," Dr. Robbins, an ichthyologist, lectured. Biology 1A was taught with a team approach, each professor teaching the part of the introductory class that matched his specialty. These fish, he said, were living examples of the evolutionary link between fins and appendages. Researchers hypothesized that when catfish were trapped in small pools by receding tides, they used their fins like legs to move when their pools dried out.

As I watched these dark, velvety bottom dwellers toddle about at the bottom of a small, light blue plastic swimming pool in the lab, I tried coming to terms with the fact that they were clever. I was used to seeing them breaded, lying inertly on ice under bright lights at the local Acme food store. Under duress though, catfish showed their adaptability and strength. I felt sorry for them crowded into their small, shallow, plastic world.

"Echinoderms, such as sea urchins, were another link," Dr. Holgrem claimed, the specialist on invertebrates. We humans share a chemical with these radially symmetrical invertebrates, one that cannot be found in any other living creature. I always thought this odd, given the huge disparity in form, function, and habitat between those spiny ones and us, but this relationship also intrigued me. We were shirttail siblings. Biochemical kin.

To get a better grip on all the new information coming at me, I resorted to Isaac Asimov's book *The Human Body* and read it secretly at the small table in the rear corner on the second floor of the university library. It was anathema for a science major to be caught reading a popular writer who covered material I should already know. I needed background, though, in order to understand the academic material. He wrote that in all human embryos, at one point in their development, gill slits form in the neck, which disappear as the fetus develops. This fact floored me. Humans with gill slits! Biologists believe that humans, in evolving from sea creatures, were the end result of a long evolutionary line of gradual complexification. So this, I marveled, was the story of how we came to be. Still, I felt unsatisfied, my deeper question unanswered.

The sexuality lectures left me puzzled. Generally, there were two types of reproduction, sexual and asexual. For the longest time, this distinction baffled me. Suddenly sexuality was a matter of gametes and diploid and haploid numbers. The sex happened when the cell went from haploid to diploid, from a single set of chromosomes to a double. But what was sexual about that? Then there was hermaphroditism. Sexuality was much more complicated than I thought. Mitosis, meiosis, how to keep track of it all? When the moon and tides dictated, a whole coral reef exploded its eggs into the water, fertilization external. Mobile larvae settled into sessile forms, the ones that don't move. In another twist, starfish regenerated from shed appendages. I couldn't keep up.

In bio lab, we were learning about radial symmetry. To my mind, it was the essence of perfection. The globed ones—sea urchins, sand dollars, sea anemones—spheres of certainty. No matter which way they are halved, the two slices are identical mirrors of one another as isomers in organic chemistry are mirror images. These types of creatures generally have a singular opening at the center and one large cavity for digestion and excretion. Their colors are varied and extraordinary: the deep purple, almost black, of echinoderm spines; the pale pink tentacles of a rose anemone, radiating from a central gold disk; the blue-pink opalescent globe of the moon jellyfish. Their form simple but elegant. Radial symmetry is balance, circularity. With bilaterally symmetrical organisms, like people, left and right halves resemble each other, but if halved at the waist, for example, top and bottom don't match. Humans have an uncanny way of throwing everything out of kilter. Humans complicate things.

Jim seemed cool, a scuba diver with beaucoup equipment and a very fancy diver's watch. His father was a doctor back in the Midwest and had bought him a Camaro for his high school graduation. I happened to sit next to him one day in bio class and liked his sarcastic sense of humor and his sweet smile. He was a big guy, about six feet, with broad shoulders and straight dirty blonde hair on a head that was small in relation to his body. This physical oddity intrigued me. He earned money on the weekend by scuba diving for lost golf balls in a pond at a nearby golf club. In one hour he retrieved over a hundred balls. Those golfers were pretty bad.

One day he asked me to see his apartment after class. I wasn't worried. It was broad daylight, and I imagined we'd have lunch together. Soon after we got there though, he showed me his room and started kissing me, nudging me toward the bed. He tugged at my shorts and fell onto me, an enormous weight. Suddenly, he did a 180-degree reversal and was sucking me before I could even register what was happening. I was in shock. His erect prick was now in my face. "Suck me," he directed. I opened my mouth. His dick was huge, and I could hardly breathe. Every once in a while, I turned my head, drawing breath. The seal had been overcome by the Orca.

I blamed myself. How naïve to think his invitation to see his apartment was innocent. I gave the wrong signal by agreeing to go. My fury boiled beneath the surface. In Jim's mind, he had done nothing wrong, it seemed, since he continued to call. I let the phone ring. I buried myself in my studies. Bodies brought trouble. Bodies laid one open to attack. Bodies are raped.

Darwin's theory of natural selection nagged at me. According to the laws of science, it seemed that my existence went against nature. Natural selection chose to discontinue me shortly after I was born, but humans intervened. Was I not then unnatural? In the seventies, Darwin had the total say on evolution, at least at the University of Miami. Only the creationists, who the scientific community shunned, questioned the wisdom of the theory described in popular terms as "the survival of the fittest." Altruism as a phenomenon directing natural selection was not discussed. I looked at myself as unfit—a weak link in the chain of evolution, a being that by virtue of my near-fatal illness had diminished the integrity of the species as a whole. From an evolutionary standpoint, I was at the bottom of the pile. I should have been allowed to die, I often thought. I was outside nature, in a category of my own—an anomaly, an aberration, a mutation. How did I fit into God's plan?

Within the world of biology, the lab was where I felt most at home. The counters were set up with trays of dead specimens. Microscopes at various locations focused on slides of potato cells, leaf cells, and a multitude of microbes in water. One corner of the lab presented the life cycle of ferns; another that of mosses. Students moved from station to station, answering questions and filling in diagrams to complete lab reports.

Dissection was a major lab activity—wielding scalpels, cutting tissue—

my kind of thing. Slipping a blade between the shells of a bivalve, severing the muscular knobs that held them shut so the organs within could be easily identified. We cut into octopi, crabs, abalone. Cutting was second nature, familiar.

In high school anatomy and physiology class, I was dubbed "The Assassin." Dr. Saglimbene required that we dissect a cat. The class was divided into four groups, each gathered around a pan in which a stiff feline lay. Ours was a tabby, pumpkin-colored. When Dr. S. asked for volunteers, for some reason, my classmates turned to me. As my buddy, Rocco, held the cat's body, I sliced at its chest. To my surprise, the body was stone hard. Try as I might, the blade would not go in. "Let me try it," Rocco suggested, but I ignored him, determined to penetrate. This time, I pulled the scalpel back over my shoulder and plunged. Success! I sawed my way down the chest past the gut as directed and then made two more incisions perpendicular to the original, one at the top of the cut and another at the bottom, to make the shape of an "I." "Great job!" Rocco congratulated. "Cutting is your thing!"

Each invertebrate was vulnerable and strangely beautiful, like an internal organ. Slicing into starfish, I felt close to them. The tiny white tube feet. The circulation system, a series of canals extending throughout the body in that perfect radial symmetry. The mouth on the underside of the starfish through which the stomach was expelled in order to envelop and devour prey. This mechanism was fascinating—how the stomach flew out of the mouth like a parachute opening and folding over its meal, digestive juices saturating the victim. It disgusted me but I was drawn to it, too. Much later, I learned about the manner in which my stomach was repaired—how the surgeon may have actually had to lift a section of it through the incision to the outside of my body in order to fix it. Starfish and I had something in common. At this time, though, I only sensed our connection.

During one lecture, it became clear that the stomach was more than what it seemed; it had a past, a developmental history that my professor traced back to the early coelenterates—primordial, sessile organisms whose digestive cavities, or coeloms, resembled the shape of a tulip. Cells specialized for breaking down food lined the inside of the flower. Digestion occurred in the same area in which excretion took place. I had never thought about an organ evolving.

In time I became fascinated with one coelenterate in particular—coral. I sought it out along the coast and researched it in the library. Coral draw in food by waving feathery frills, like tiny propellers, that surround an opening into a digestive cavity. This mode of feeding determines its life to a large degree, so in a way, immobility defines it. Coral cannot run from predators. Parrotfish nibble on it and divers break off hunks, yet the coral can do nothing. In order to eat, they must stay put. So much then of the lives of coral, it seemed to me, was up to chance. In a similar way, my stomach defined my limitations. I did not choose to have a dysfunctional stomach. In order to digest food and hence survive, surgery was a must. It was what happened to me. I was what happened to me.

Starfish, barnacles, clams, octopi, and sharks, killed and prepared long before the semester started, crowded the shelves and counters of the biology labs. It was quite another thing, however, to carry out the killing oneself. For the lesson about the nervous system, I was required to kill a frog. I picked up the needle without hesitation. Had I procrastinated even a second, I would not have been able to jab the frog's head as the instructor directed and watch its legs kick though it was technically dead. Apparently, even after death, electricity, created by an exchange of ions, still moves positive charges across muscle tissue. The experience was horrifying. I can still hear the students' whoops and whoas as one frog jumped right off the lab counter. I still feel the moment when my pin punctured the frog's skull and entered something soft. Bio lab was no longer where I wanted to be.

I was always attracted to the darkest part of the ocean—the underwater trenches where creatures live without light under tons of pressure. A place where ancient armored fish called coelacanths still swim; where only submersibles or underwater cameras venture; where creatures make their own light. Inaccessible places where sound waves send back information, and undersea fissures spew magma, the water bubbling and chaotic as molten rock meets freezing water. Life lives in the darkest, coldest places, miles below the surface in unimaginable conditions. I was fascinated by that place called the abyss.

Marine creatures go to great lengths to adapt to this extreme—a lantern hanging over a mouth; a long row of bioluminescent dots lining an underbelly; wide mouths with long needle-like teeth and scales like armor. Under the weight of all that water, sea cucumbers suck food off the sea floor, and crabs and spiny lobsters comb boulders for nourishment. Bacteria feed from the sea floor layered with detritus, organic matter that piles up. No matter how difficult the conditions, living beings find ways to survive.

In the abyss, creatures take advantage of everything whether it's a fecal pellet falling from the surface miles above or a chunk of wood thrown from the deck of a ship. Sea life congregates around thermal vents, openings or fissures in the earth's crust from which lava flows. Heat draws a select crowd of grazers.

Most animals survive by rising to the surface waters during the day, where they feed. Whole communities composed of millions of organisms—shrimp, fish, squid, and jellyfish—ascend, returning to the depths by night. These schools are so thick that they disrupt sonar readings; hence, they are referred to as deep scattering layers. From these organisms drop what is called marine snow, waste matter that feeds bottom dwellers with a continual rain of nourishment. Sponges, lobsters, crabs, sea worms, sea stars, sea urchins, and radiolaria all live where life seems forsaken.

At the beginning of my second semester, something from the deep washed ashore that threatened to drag me into the undertow and pull me beyond reach. Abby Finegold was one of my suitemates in the dorm my first semester. Sherry, my Resident Adviser, warned me not to get involved with her, but I did not listen. Ostensibly what drew me was the drama of her life—her nightly arguments with her mother and her boyfriend—and my wish to save her. Who could help but hear her screaming into the telephone receiver and sobbing in her room? In my family, we smoldered in silence like coals. In any event, Abby and I ended up in a paddy wagon one afternoon bound for the Miami Dade Jail.

Abby and I had driven to the mall in her white Corvette. At a department store, I spotted Abby stuffing shorts and tank tops into a satchel in the shopping basket. She saw me noticing and winked. Why is she shoplifting? She's rich enough to afford whatever she wants.

But as I saw the amount of stuff she was taking, I got jealous. I wanted stuff, too. I couldn't afford more than the one bathing suit. I tucked a black pair of shorts into my bag and a turquoise tank top. On cue from Abby, we headed out the door. Two male undercover security guards raced from the store, yelling, "Stop right there!"

We did. Stan, our lawyer, told us later that all we had to do was drop the bags. The law required that we be apprehended in the store with the merchandise on our person. I remember being surprised by his comments. After all, we had committed a crime. Since he was a friend of the Finegold family, shouldn't he have lectured us about not stealing? Looking back, I am astounded by my naiveté.

I'll never forget the sound of the barred gate opening on the second floor of the jail. When the guard pulled a lever, a deafening clank roared down the hall. I felt as if I had died and been taken to an interim place where my fate would be determined, Heaven or Hell.

I was eighteen. The cell was dark as it was already night. Getting fingerprinted, booked and strip searched by a female guard who made me stand astride and bend over so she could look into the crack of my butt and then run her hand between my legs, took awhile. I felt defeated and helpless. How much lower could my life go? In my cell, I was warned by an inmate not to sit on the "toilet"—a hole in the floor—or I'd get crabs. "Don't use the sink either if ya know what's good for ya," a disembodied voice called from beyond the wall.

In my cell kneeled a Hispanic woman whom Abby and I had sat with in the paddy wagon, an agonizing ride during which Abby frantically tried to hide the marijuana she had stashed in her makeup bag. She ended up shoving it somewhere behind her seat. That's all I needed—to be arrested for possession of drugs, too! The woman had also been arrested for shoplifting, in her case, a plastic hairbrush. Abby avoided getting locked up. Later I learned that she had called her family lawyer who drove immediately to Dade County Jail to pay her bail and chauffer her home. Abby was free now, and only the Hispanic woman and I were left behind bars.

The woman knelt on the floor of the cell all night, her forearms resting on a table as she rocked back and forth, praying. I didn't know the Spanish words but heard the exhortation and understood the word "Jesus." At one point, I lost patience with her crying and mumbling. In English, I told her to stop, raising my hands to pantomime, but she wouldn't even look my way. Her dark form swayed in the dim light. Her voice pierced the air. In the morning, I left her behind, though the sounds of her desperate prayers to a God I had long since renounced still haunted me. How unjust the world was. More than that though, she symbolized my imprisoned soul, trapped in the notion that I was not whole and never would be.

Phil, Abby's lawyer, was a con man. I did not know this when I approached him for help the day after my release from jail. Abby had secured his counsel for me but, as I was to learn, there would be more than a price.

His fee was fifteen hundred dollars, he informed me. I was shocked. Naively, I didn't see why I had to pay. Shoplifting had been Abby's idea. Since Phil was the family lawyer, why shouldn't they foot the bill? I told him that I didn't have the money but would be working all summer and could pay him come fall. Phil cut me a deal. Either I paid then or I could pay another way.

He motioned me to him and pointed to his lap. I felt unsteady as I approached his darkly stained desk. Sitting where he directed, I felt his hand on the small of my back. I focused on the chandelier in the center of the ceiling, a particular crystal teardrop hanging at the periphery, as he rubbed. I cannot recall what he actually said, but I understood the price if I could not come up with the money.

As he ran his hand up and down my bare arm, he told me that the judge would take a bribe and that this money I owed him would, in part, be used for this purpose. The Finegolds owned a furniture store and the judge liked leather chairs and couches. Besides, the judge was his fishing buddy, not to worry. He squeezed my wrist and told me he would see me in court in two weeks. At the door, I smiled meekly.

Along the rugged coast of Japan, a lantern hangs from a Shinto shrine perched on a cliff's edge, blessing and paying homage to the AMA divers, women of great bravery, strength, and endurance. These women dive sixty feet into the cold seas surrounding Japan without scuba equipment to pry abalone and other delicacies from the rocks of the sea floor. To me they seem to defy the odds as they pull themselves to those depths, enough air left for collecting food and ascending. Naked from the waist up, white-creamed goggled faces, knives tucked into their tight diving shorts, each woman procures nearly thirty pounds of seafood a day. They are pulled to the surface by ropes tied to their waists. Midday, AMA divers crowd around a fire and warm themselves, chatting and eating their lunches in preparation for their afternoon dives. These were women who penetrated the depths and survived.

The first person I saw in the lobby of my dorm when I arrived the following fall was Abby. University fees and book costs used up much of the money I saved at my summer job, working as a blueprint copier at Graver Water Company on Route 22 in New Jersey. I was resigned to my fate. I would have to fuck Phil.

"Have you spoken to Phil?" I asked.

"Don't ask," Abby said.

My eyebrows flew up. I stood arms akimbo, staring, needing an answer.

"Concrete shoes," Abby said, "Mafia stuff. Leave it alone." I stood, mouth agape, as Abby disappeared into the elevator. Phil had been murdered. Relief flooded in. That was the last time I saw Abby Finegold. I moved to the Honors Dormitory, back on track. Back to being perfect girl.

Nigricans

There is, one knows not what sweet mystery about this sea, whose gently awful stirrings seem to speak of some hidden soul beneath. —Herman Melville

I found my soul mate in Pennekamp Underwater State Park. Each student in Biology 100 was required to turn in an algae collection accompanied by a key, a written guide identifying each specimen. Each organism had to be sketched and keyed. Drawing was no problem nor was collecting. I enjoyed illustrating and loved snorkeling. I had seen photos of many reef creatures in magazines and textbooks, so it was thrilling to actually meet them for the first time. Some though were entirely new to me. I came to admire acetabularia, a golden cup attached to a long, slender stem that floated in the currents, like a kite. But Nigricans, a chocolate brown, double-lobed, heart-shaped alga of rich velvet, like the robe of a queen, stole my heart. Both algae were solitary growers, securing themselves onto single rocks with holdfasts, raptor-like claws. They filtered seawater for food, swaying all day in curtains of golden green sunlight and all night in deep purple shadows.

Amid sheets of light along the side of an underwater trench, a Nigricans perched majestically atop a rock, anchored by her holdfast. Her thick, dark brown lobes glittered with a soft, gold sheen as she waved gracefully, dancing in the currents. I kicked over to her and hovered, mesmerized by her beauty—perhaps the most magnificent organism that I had ever seen. Her presence gave me a sense of something deep inside—the reality of my own glorious beauty.

Greedily, I snatched the Nigricans for my collection, committing the same crime as hundreds of other bio majors, the probable reason for the temporary closure of the park at a future point so that the algae could regenerate. Then, I grabbed the acetabularia.

I did not know that years later back at home in New Jersey, having given up my dream of becoming a marine biologist, I would come upon my algae collection in the closet, the water root beer brown and the organisms blackened and flaccid. Formaldehyde would not preserve their perfect forms as I had hoped, and it would no longer be possible to distinguish one species from another. Where was the Nigricans I loved amid the layers, I would wonder. Where was that glittering, soft gold sheen?

By the end of the first semester in my second year at the university, I had made the Dean's List, studying weekends in the lounge overlooking the lake, and had met a whole new group of bio major friends: Rory, Melody, Sara, and Hank. They urged me to apply for the Everglades Water Chemistry Field Project, funded by the National Science Foundation for the coming summer, so that we could spend the vacation together. One chilly January morning, I sat on a bench outside the math classrooms, filling out the application.

I had procrastinated and the pressure was on to turn it in that day. The goal of the project was to determine the cause of the sudden deaths of hundreds of fish—fish kills. The political subtext of the grant was to save the Everglades—a slow-moving, shallow river that flowed through grasses, forests, and other subtropical plant communities—from the building of the Jetport, an international airport. In some parts of the Glades, it was already under construction.

Why should they pick me, I wondered as my pen hovered in confusion over the blank space. I was no science genius like Sara or brilliant like Melody, who won a full scholarship to U of M. I could not think of a thing to write, except to say that I wanted to help save the Everglades. On the application, I mentioned having read *Silent Spring* in high school and being aware of the danger of the cracking of eggs.

When I heard that I was chosen to be a member of the National Science Foundation team, I thought there had been some mistake. The amateur research scientist identification card with my name on it that arrived in my mailbox set all doubts to rest. I was chosen to help save the Glades!

That spring semester, just before the project kicked in, I hit a major snag in genetics lab. I couldn't make any sense of fruit flies and their wings. The small squadron of black bugs lay in formation on the paper under my microscope. Adjusting the focus, I noted the type of wings of each fly: two identical or one wing smaller, vestigial? I marked the results in groups of five, four vertical lines bisected with a slash, the way my grammar school gym teacher kept score for kick ball. What equation would make sense of that chaos of numbers? Applying algebra was beyond me. I had worked hard to earn a "C" in high school algebra and trig. In genetics, math sunk me. I sat like a heavy chunk of lead at the bottom of a sea of calculations. I was no AMA diver. Panicked, I flailed my arms and legs in an effort to surface.

I stole Antonia's lab reports. My roommate kept her genetics lab reports, papers gridded with light blue boxes like tiny cages, in the trunk at the foot of her bed. Each week, I copied her completed assignment by hand and returned it to the trunk, turning in my copy for a grade. We had the same TA for genetics lab though at different times. Fortunately, he did not check for plagiarism. I risked getting kicked out of school, but the grade mattered more. Graduate school depended on it.

Across campus from the Honors Dorm, I hid in a cubicle at the rear of my old dorm's study room and modified Antonia's work by adding more details to a graph, rewording the interpretation of the data, and manipulating the numbers. The ratios would be the same, which is what mattered; arithmetic I knew. At first the goal had been to avoid flunking; I would copy only enough to pass. But as I manipulated Antonia's calculations and interpretations, I realized how excellent her work was and that I could get an "A." I began to incorporate everything.

One morning on my way to the infamous cubicle, the most recent of Antonia's gems tucked into my notebook, I spotted her coming toward me on the wide sandy path, heading back toward our apartment. I froze.

"Hey," I called, trying to sound natural, "I thought you were going to class."

"Oh, I just decided the heck with it all," Antonia said, "I'm going fishing. Got to catch the big one!" She looked over at her friend and laughed.

I panicked. Had she found me out or was this just her Midwestern sense of humor? "C'mon," I pleaded.

"I told you. I'm going fishing," she replied, gleefully, shifting the weight of her books. "It's going to be a whopper!"

"Oh, shit!" I exclaimed, staging frustration. "I forgot my textbook."

"To hell with it," Antonia said. "Come fishing with us."

"Right!" I said, sprinting down the path back to the dorm.

Just inside the door, I paused. My heart was racing. I willed myself to proceed deliberately and quickly. She was just down the path and surely would return to her room. As I opened the trunk and slipped the lab report back into place, a pain stabbed my chest. Never again, I vowed.

"My class was canceled, silly!" Antonia told me, throwing her books down on the couch.

There was no fish to catch; she hadn't a clue. A few days later, I was at it again.

That summer I moved to a room in the SAE house, ironically the same fraternity I had fled over a year ago during my first weeks at school. The blond boys had left for the summer and rent was cheap. Several of the students chosen for the Everglades Project were rooming there. In one sense, I suppose I was doing penance for cheating—residing in a small, dark, windowless room with a tiny fridge and a small bathroom. In reality, I just didn't want to see anyone; I felt so bad about myself. Cheating from Antonia's notes had affected me deeply. Were the project leaders aware that they had a loser on their hands? My life was a series of cycles of climbs to great places and grave dives from grace. A dream baby/a burden baby. A good baby/ an ugly baby. Everything good turned sour.

Each night I retired to my cell to read books—*Deliverance, Frannie and Zooey, Notes From Underground*. If friends knocked on my door, I plugged my ears and kept on reading. Bent on finishing *Anna Karenina* by the end of the summer, I was living the life of a monk, cloistered from society.

Two weeks into the summer, Melody, also chosen to work on the Glades project, asked me to rent an apartment with her on Red Road, a short bike ride from the university. At first, I argued for my ascetic existence. She merely laughed, telling me how much more comfortable I'd be if we shared a place. Finally, I consented. Perhaps I had suffered enough. At the corner of Frat Row and Palm Drive, she picked up me and all my worldly goods—stereo, bicycle, and trunk full of books and clothes—and whisked us off to a promising new life.

Saving the Glades was more than a full-time job. Weekday mornings, while the searing sun was still low in the sky, Melody and I took off in her car, heading for a site along the elaborate system of canals in south Florida. We checked a new one each day. These waterways, built to reroute water from the Glades in order to serve the residents of the new surrounding housing tracts, were included in our study. Kevin, our project mate, had rigged up a system whereby Mel and I could run the Millipore Filter right off the battery in her car. We thought we were pretty cool, measuring chlorophyll on site—a new phenomenon in ecology.

Weekends, we often camped out in the swamp itself, taking water samples every two hours day and night. Days were blindingly sunny with few places to take shade. The water we walked in was sometimes over 100 degrees. In every direction though, the beauty of the glades stretched magnificently: acres of green sawgrass; dense thickets of cypress swamp; blue sky and white cumulus clouds, so tall, dense with moisture, and close to the earth, like clipper ships of old sailing the waves of air.

The night sky was vast, often a deep, uninterrupted, ultramarine blue. Insect sounds were deafening, hundreds of millions of tiny creatures, alternately creating euphony and cacophony—certainly a one-of-a kind symphony. One night a bug dropped onto my shoulder that barely fit into my empty Marlboro pack. It had giant pincers and body armor; I brought it to show my fellow researchers. They wouldn't have believed me had I not shown it to them.

Sometimes the Glades were dangerous. Once at two in the morning as we paddled our raft packed with the water chemistry set out into the water hole, Melody noticed two small golden globes hovering near the sample site. The only entry in our log that night was "Alligator!"

Every Monday, Mel and I brought our test tubes to the Rosenstiel School of Marine Science, the U of M grad school, and blasted open the chloroplasts with the cell sonifier so that we could measure the chlorophyll. We became familiar faces on Virginia Key. Actually, we did almost everything together, taking in movies on the weekend and spending time at her parents' home. That summer, if I bumped into friends when I wasn't with Melody, "Where's Mel?" was the first question out of their mouths.

I met Mitch, one of those Greek god-looking types with dark curly hair and green eyes, when Melody and I were picking up a load of dry ice at the airport. A new grad student at the marine lab, he was searching for his crate of frogs at the cargo pickup platform. Brazenly, I suggested a welcome-to-

Florida tour of our beloved "river of grass" in the coming week.

At one stop along Alligator Alley, the main road through the Everglades, we discovered an abandoned Seminole Indian village. I stood on Mitch's shoulders in order to get a look over the wall. It was eerie. The village was intact but not a soul was in sight. Suddenly it occurred to me that the floor of the village seemed to be moving. I stared at the wall opposite to get my bearings. On its surface crawled hundreds if not thousands of huge yellow grasshoppers with large brown spots. They seethed on every surface. I felt nauseous.

Mitch was intrigued. I gave him a leg up so that he could see for himself. Thrilled with the sight, he convinced me to go in with him, assuring me that he would carry me on his shoulders if I freaked out. Once inside the village walls with Mitch, I felt afraid. Could they bite? Would they crawl up my legs? Statue-like, I stood next to the fence while Mitch explored.

Oddly, the grasshoppers ignored me, going about their business. As they sprang from one side of the yard to the other, I ducked from sheer reflex. Grasshoppers bypassed my feet, heading in one direction, treating me as if I were an aspect of the landscape. I began to relax enough to notice that the grasshoppers on the walls were copulating, fucking up a storm. There were mountings with legs at critical angles. And there were Mitch and I in the midst of it all. At one point, he smiled seductively at me; I smiled back shyly.

Later that afternoon as we were soaking in a waterhole, trying to cool off, he swam over and reached for me. We kissed, and he pressed his hard dick against me. I was uncomfortable, my sacrum shoved up against some jagged projection. I was interested but bothered by the fact that I hardly knew him. When his grip slipped, I swam away.

That evening, as we kissed good-bye in his car outside my apartment, he asked to stay over. I told him I had a roommate and didn't want to disturb her.

"You do have your own bedroom, don't you?" he asked sarcastically.

I turned away. "Some other time." He never called again, and I did not call him. I wanted a boyfriend, not a quick fuck. Melody had started dating and on weekends, we were spending less time together. Where was that person with whom I could open myself?

The nautilus is the jewel of the depths. One of the most beautiful and mysterious creatures on the planet, not only is its shell a work of art, delicate and intricate, but it is an architectural marvel with its staircase of steps circling within. Unperturbed by the enormous weight of water, the nautilus generally lives at great depths. Once a year though, this animal ascends within a range of five hundred to a thousand feet from the surface, looking for a mate. At this time, the creature is vulnerable to capture. This always seemed very romantic to me—the way the nautilus risks its life to find a partner.

A blind date with a law student friend of a friend was a desperate attempt to find a boyfriend. At that point, I just had to go out with someone. Anyone! Back at his apartment after dinner, he insisted that I draw on him with pink lipstick as he stripped down to his underpants and lay on his belly on his bed. I drew a circle or two on his shoulder and a long line down his bumpy spine, then told him that I was ready to go home. He was, to my mind, a nutcase. Why couldn't I find someone suitable? Everyone else seemed to be finding a mate. Why was I alone?

I retreated to spending time at what bio majors called "the shacks," the old science building, tucked into a grove of palm trees, hidden from view by green fronds. Rory, one of my Everglades research buddies, had kindly made me a copy of his key, which he had gotten from a graduate student friend of his, Larry. I created a routine for myself. In the evenings after work, I swam laps at the Olympic-sized pool, eavesdropping on lessons that a coach was teaching an Olympic hopeful, and tried out some new techniques.

Afterward, I picked up a sandwich at the cafeteria and walked over to the shacks. I felt comforted by the sight of the old wooden structures, the peeling paint and the roof sloping at an odd angle, a few of its shingles missing. The ultra-modern biology building, a short walk away, was steel and glass, lit with fluorescent lights. By contrast the shacks were illumined by softly glowing bulbs screwed into low hanging, green-shaded lamps, and the counters and floors were made of wood. Orchids, hanging from slabs of brown bark, specimens of Dr. Fontaine's, welcomed me as I unlocked the main door, and the steady bubbling of Dr. Holgrem's snail aquariums comforted me. I often passed Lance, a grad student, on his way out. He seemed archetypical with his full red beard and ruddy, weathered skin, and a chameleon, green during the summer, draped over his shoulder.

One lab I avoided was Dr. Keefering's after encountering a live horseshoe crab in a tub containing an inch of water. The front portion of its shell had been cut away and its eyes wired to technology. I had heard about his study of the horseshoe crab's simple eyes in order to understand our more complex ones and knew that horseshoe crabs were ideal specimens for this purpose because of their primitive origins, but to actually see it—I gasped, grabbing the edge of the counter, afraid I'd sink down onto my knees. Thank God I was alone. I blinked back the tears and made for the door.

Each night at Larry's desk, I drank a glass of red wine and nibbled at my sandwich as I read *The Voyage of the Beagle* or Lily's book about the intelligence of dolphins. It was extremely dark out at the shacks, the light of my desk lamp the only brightness. No curtains shielded the windows, and no public lighting lit the walkways alongside the offices. I brushed away my fears, unwilling to accept that being a woman made me any more vulnerable than a guy. Even so, I jumped at every little noise, constantly peeking over the pages to make sure that I was not being watched from the darkness.

At the shacks, I often caught snatches of conversation between grad students. Some were suspicious of Dr. Rosen. Rumor was that he had begun a private environmental consulting firm, slanting research data in favor of developers. When a real estate company needed an environmental impact study before building on property bordering the Everglades, good ole Doc Rosen was available for a consult. Outraged students claimed that he was using university facilities to carry out this private practice. As I watched his graduate assistant wash all his lab equipment and file his consulting company's data, I realized that saving the Glades was a lot more complicated than I imagined.

One Sunday afternoon, Rory and I were in charge of monitoring the canals on the east side of the Glades. I liked him. He was in his final year as a biology major at U of M and had already been accepted to graduate school somewhere in the state of Washington, far away. By this time, both of us were grungy and grimy from a weekend of living in a van, so he suggested that we mutiny and drive to Dr. Jergen's house a few miles from the collection site to shower. He was away for the summer, and Rory had the key to his home.

At Dr. J's, Rory made us coffee, eggs, and toast. What luxury after sleeping and eating in the university science van parked on the bank of a South Florida canal! Since we were both Ayn Rand fans, we got so wrapped up in a discussion of *Atlas Shrugged* that by the time we noticed the clock, we were late for the next scheduled water sample.

As soon as we pulled up to the site, we were astonished to see dozens of dead fish floating on the surface of the canal. We had missed the fish kill—the reason for the Glades project in the first place! I whipped out the water chemistry set, shoved the probes into the water, and jotted down meter readings. Rory took notes concerning cloud cover, water level, and vegetation. The oxygen reading reported a steep decrease. The fish's blue gills told of a lack of oxygen. Rory called the county flood control department and discovered that the closing of the floodgates, one of which was within twenty feet, occurred only a half-hour previous to our arrival. Could the elaborate system of floodgates built by the Army Corps of Engineers have had something to do with the fish kills? Perhaps the sudden closure caused rapid oxygen depletion, though we couldn't be sure the fish hadn't died earlier since we were late.

We fudged the report, stating that we had arrived at the fish kill within minutes and noting the floodgate as a possible culprit. I felt awful. I blamed Rory for wooing me away from the site in the first place though I realized I had consented to go. Once again, I had made the wrong choice. Same old, same old—I was unreliable at the core.

Toward the end of the summer, Melody, Rory, Sara, and I tagged along with the University of Miami's graduate ornithology class on a trip to the Dry Tortugas, islands off the coast of Florida. At midnight we boarded a cattle boat and the next day we arrived at Fort Jefferson, the unofficial birding capital of the Tortugas and the place where Dr. Samuel Alexander Mudd, an accomplice of the man who assassinated President Lincoln, had been imprisoned. Much of the fort still stood, walls rising from rock along a third of the island's shoreline.

Just off the dock, a pelican captured my heart. A vestigial wing, tiny and undeveloped, clung close to the bird's body. The pelican could not fly. As soon as I saw it floating alongside the pier, a deep bond took hold. Apparently, the pelican had lived there all its life. Visitors kept it fed, especially a kind captain who regularly moored his shrimp boat at the dock. I felt moved by everyone's attempts to keep it alive. I took a photo of it, floating in the teal blue jewel of water—a robust, healthy bird but for one stunted wing.

As the Glades project came to an end, I felt uncertain about whether to continue at the University of Miami. Maybe it was the controversy surrounding Dr. Rosen's consulting practice or what Sara had told me during a visit to her family's home in Delaware. At the orchid conference that she attended in the Florida Keys midsummer, Dr. Fontaine, married with two young children, knocked on her door nightly, insisting that she have sex with him, which she refused. After two years studying ecology, I was jaded. Intrigues, scandals and shady deals prevailed. The cracking of eggs seemed irremediable.

One night during the visit, I hung out in Sara's basement, watching her and her father prepare gifts for friends of the family. On the big table saw, he cut wood for frames while she placed the most beautiful dead butterflies onto thick pieces of cotton. These specimens, the ones she had been studying in Venezuela with Dr. Jergens over winter break, were centered under glass and framed. Each butterfly was huge, five inches wide by three, and one of two types: lemon yellow with brown circles marking the lower wings or iridescent turquoise, wings edged with black. There must have been at least thirty of these dead beauties lying in cotton coffins. Had she captured and killed them for presents? I could not find the courage to ask. More and more, it seemed that biology was the study of the dead and not the living.

All summer, I looked forward to taking the introductory course in embryology in the fall. The class required lots of memorization and illustration, both of which I was good at. A friend showed me his notebooks of meticulous drawings he had made in colored pencil, thin lines emanating from each curled embryo and pointing to a long scientific word. I craved understanding the development of the embryos in those jars. That was the class for me.

But I never got to trace the early stages of life. I left U of M after my summer Everglades project, returning home to live in my old bedroom. I just didn't believe myself smart enough to be a scientist, so why keep fooling myself? Besides, I couldn't even scuba dive!

I had taken a crash course my first semester at college—a weekend in Key Largo where by the end of three days of intensive swimming, studying, practicing scuba in a pool, and ocean diving, we were to get our diving certifications. But I had flunked the test!

In the doff and don test, where you remove your diving gear at the deepest part of the pool, fly to the surface, take a breath, and return to clear the regulator, breathe tank air, and hoist the scuba gear back on, I couldn't clear the regulator. Water dumped into my lungs and I flew to the surface, choking and coughing my way up. I swam poolside and sat clutching my knees, shaking on the edge, where my instructor ordered me to "get back on the horse." I shook my head, waving him off, and never resumed the test.

He allowed me to take the ocean dive the next day anyway, conferring the license on me despite flunking the pool test. The failure though had stripped me of confidence. As I descended forty feet underwater, the pressure on my ears was enormous. When I neared the sandy bottom, no other diver was near. I panicked. The sound of breathing through a regulator, the dependence on the air tube wrapping over my shoulder, the aloneness in an alien world, the constriction of the tanks strapped to my back, the necessity of deliberate movements slowing time.

Desperate, I looked up. There were my fellow divers hovering twenty feet above me. Relief! I chided myself for my foolishness. As they descended, I relaxed enough to enjoy the maze-like surfaces of huge brain corals and the long, chocolate-brown arms of staghorn coral.

I knew though as soon as I surfaced that I was done with diving. I'd brushed against something primordial deep inside me, something terrifying. But like a shark "sleeping" in underwater, spring-fed caves, it was better left undisturbed. Best to let danger sleep, narcotized by super-oxygenated water pumping over gill slits.

Back home in New Jersey, I removed everything from my bulletin board—the photos of scuba divers, marine creatures, and Jacques Cousteau—and pinned up the photo of the pelican with one vestigial wing.

≈≈≈

Twenty years old, a dropout of the University of Miami, I was living again with my parents, working at the hospital as a ward clerk. Maybe becoming a doctor would be more suitable. I spent a lot of time reflecting on my situation.

As a girl, I struggled with reading and algebra; as a young woman, fruit flies and sex. Why couldn't I read faster? Why was algebra an unlocked code? Why were the fruit flies a mystery? Why was finding a boyfriend so difficult?

Maybe I had never been completely put back together. Even though I could digest food and was basically healthy, *I didn't work.* At my core, I worried that perhaps once the body was broken into at such an early age, it could not really ever mend, like Humpty Dumpty. How horrible that story was to me as a child. The picture of that awful broken egg. There he lay, shards of white shell scattered about, suspenders limp, pants filled with eggshell. Was there no one who could repair him?

After working all day at the hospital, I took up the work of biology in the evenings. My old high school boyfriend and bio-buddy, Steven, got me a shark from the biology department at Rutgers University, where he was a student. His class had just finished studying shark anatomy, and there were some specimens left over. I bought a spiffy dissection kit in a royal blue case with shiny scalpels, clamps, and tweezers and set up the red-covered card table in my bedroom. "Happy cutting!" Steven joked as he handed over the shark in a plastic bag along with an illustrated manual, which directed a novice through an ordered exploration of the fish's body. I lay the bag, stinking of formaldehyde, in an aluminum pan and wrapped it all up with another plastic bag.

I was excited about dissecting the shark but scared, too. Without the help of a lab instructor, could I do it right? Flipping through the pages of the lab manual, the digestive organs chapter caught my eye. I propped the book open to the directions for entering the abdomen of the shark and began. Pressing my scalpel into the thick, gray carcass of the shark, the skin gave way. Cutting calmed me. I liked holding the razor-sharp edge to skin and making a precise slice. Unknown territory beckoned. I was on the trail of something—a discovery just beyond the tip of the blade as if on the verge of finding something I'd lost. As the manual directed, I cut a square flap into the shark's side, folded it back, and pinned it with a hook.

As diagrammed, the pouch of the stomach revealed itself. Very slowly and carefully, I slit the bag, which was quite tough. To my surprise, there were three undigested fish inside! The lab book had not noted that I might actually encounter something in the sac! With tweezers, I extracted the fish, one by one, and set them on a paper towel. Undigested, they were perfect, flat oval shapes; only the fins and the eyes had disintegrated. I felt a sense of triumph. I had made my way into the stomach and figured out what the contents were!

My mother knocked on my door, wondering if I wanted a snack. "Look," I said, pointing to the fish. "These were in the shark's stomach!"

She sidled up to the table. "They look like sand dabs," she said in a matter-of-fact way, "your father's favorite." With that, she turned and headed for the door. I was floored. Didn't she get it? These were fish I had excavated from the stomach of a shark! "Got to get Dad a beer before the commercial's over."

To hell with Dad and his beer, I wanted to say. I felt completely deflated, my excitement dashed. Why didn't she care about what I'd found? I'd excavated a shark stomach. Couldn't she see how important this was?

I looked back down at the brown ovals. There they lay on the paper towel, one next to the other, slightly overlapping, like cards in a flush. Maybe they weren't so special. Should I throw them out? But the shark didn't seem whole without them. I slipped the fish back into the stomach—they fit so perfectly—and wrapped the shark back up in plastic for the night.

I couldn't get those undigested fish out of my mind. It didn't seem fair that the shark's life had been wrested in the middle of a meal to satisfy someone's curiosity, that its young life had been interrupted. Mutilating the shark further just didn't seem right. The next day, I carried the shark in its plastic coffin to the garbage can on the side of our house and tossed it in.

～～～

Melody lured me back to Florida. Maybe I still had a chance in science. I had applied to a couple of East Coast colleges but wouldn't hear until the end of the summer. Certainly, I was tired of being ordered around by pompous doctors and harried, unappreciated nurses. And at home, I felt in the way. Tolerated. My parents seemed to be biding their time until I left again. Besides, Ray, the guy I was dating, whom I had started to really like, turned to me in the car after our last date and, instead of kissing me as I anticipated, apologized, saying, "I think you should know that I'm gay."

Mel's roommate was leaving, and I could move right in. Her father would sell me his old car, and Dr. Segar, her former boss at the U of M graduate school, the Rosenstiel School on Virginia Key where we'd sonified cells for the Glades Project, would hire me as a tech level two for the Mid-Atlantic Ridge Research Project. Conveniently, Mel worked across the street at NOAA, the National Oceanographic and Atmospheric Administration. Everything was in place. Mel and I would buddy up once again.

In Dr. Segar's physical oceanography lab, I ran the atomic adsorption spectrophotometer, one of only seven in the world, a huge and costly machine that analyzed the composition of seawater. I felt honored and awed. Each year, the Rosenstiel School's research vessel embarked on a trans-Atlantic journey, collecting seawater samples at varying depths, arriving at a port in Africa far north of the previous year's destination so as to cover new territory on each journey. Hundreds of crates of plastic bottles with labels, such as M-2, C-32, Z-72, crowded the floor of the lab awaiting analysis. Dr. Segar was studying the nature of a mountain range far below the surface of the Atlantic. Perhaps it was volcanic? The hypothesis was exciting; proving it was not.

First thing in the morning, I prepared the water sample by following a formula, a recipe if you will. I recorded the weight of the samples, added chemicals, weighed again, and shook the mixture in order to fix or stabilize the seawater.

From each prepared bottle, I drew out several samples, injected them into the analyzer, and jotted the bottle numbers into a ledger. The analyzer subjected the seawater to extremely high temperatures. Because each element in the water emitted a characteristic wavelength, Dr. Segar could identify it later. He then graphed these results onto a map to show the progression of the concentrations of the different elements. In any case, trace metals were present in high numbers at points in the Atlantic Ocean that traced the north-south mountain range. The existence of these metals in waters over the Mid-Atlantic Ridge suggested the nature of the range to be volcanic, an important finding. Meanwhile, I was bored. Agitated, too. Daily, a weird lab tech level one guy stared lewdly at me as he washed test tubes.

In high school, I had imagined the life of a scientist—sitting at water's edge in khakis and swamp boots, drawing a kite bird and the surrounding flora with my colored pencils. Instead, I stood beside my trusty analyzer under glaring florescent lights each early morning until late afternoon. Measurement was our god.

While carrying out these tasks, I wore a three-quarter-length white lab coat and blue jeans, my red hair tied back into a long ponytail. Latex gloves and brown leather sandals completed the outfit, a costume that belied the seriousness of the task. I worked with meticulous care: sterilizing the injector before each immersion into the sample; injecting the sample into the analyzer with a practiced, steady motion so that no spills occurred; monitoring the level of heat blasting the seawater at temperatures that would have made toast of me; and ensuring that the stylus on the recorder touched the graph paper properly as it leapt to action, staggering across the grid in sudden peaks and troughs. The flat line announced the finish, followed by a hiss of the machine. Sample after sample, mile after mile of graph paper. The work of science was tedious.

In between sample injections, I memorized vocabulary words and tested them out on Dr. Segar and my co-workers. From my nightly readings of Ayn Rand and science fiction, I compiled lists of words, supplied them with definitions and sample sentences, and then propped this tiny spiral notepad against the side of the behemoth machine. Words like *halcyon, hiatus, sycophant, pusillanimous,* and *solipsism* filled its pages. I did this not out of a love of words or an attempt to balance art and science; I believed that I needed to improve myself, that who I was or what I was doing was never enough.

"Are you thoroughly recovered from your illness that caused a brief *hiatus* from work?" I asked Dr. Segar.

He smiled impishly, playing along with my game. "Absolutely, my dear Watson. I see you've kept the ship afloat in my 'brief hiatus' as you call it." He was English and spoke with an accent. "Your assiduousness is to be commended."

He and I had developed a polite and friendly connection. Sometimes, I stood at his office door, listening to him disparage the Nixon administration as the drama of Watergate unfolded on a tiny TV that Dr. Segar perched atop huge stacks of graph paper. He relished the humiliation of the American government. It gave him more pleasure than even I, a classic cynic, was comfortable with. I nodded, placating him. Truth be told, I paid little attention to politics. He was my boss, and I felt I had to listen.

Toward the end of summer, Dr. Segar surprised me by proposing that I be his technician for the trip to Africa that coming fall. Typically, I put a self-effacing spin on his invitation. I was the perfect tech, I supposed, meticulously carrying out his plans and posing no threat to a scientist's ego. My skills—precision, loyalty, attention to detail, and organizational acumen—none of these came to mind. Then the issue of what I believed my fundamental unreliability rattled me. How could he trust me—a screw-up—with this huge responsibility? Weighing heavily was also the fact that I'd be the only female on board. Would some scientist be banging nightly at my door? On a ship, there was nowhere to run.

My own dreams dormant, my intelligence submerged, I swam on the surface of the ocean, unable to gain access to my depths. A net trapped my sense of agency, the integrity of my core in constant question. I equivocated for weeks. In the end, my acceptance to Barnard College in New York City made my decision for me.

One Saturday, I drove myself to John Pennekamp Marine Park in the Keys, about an hour and a half south of Coral Gables, where I went snorkeling. Taking a whole day to do something pleasurable for myself was unusual for me. I remember gathering my equipment from the back of the car and feeling paralyzed with self-consciousness. I felt fat and ugly in my two-piece suit and couldn't wait to sink into the water to conceal myself. Once below the surface, I became so engrossed by an angelfish, its stripes and vivid colors, that all my feelings of shame dissolved. Completely present, I watched, marveling at the black dot near the fish's tail fin that mimicked an eye, nature's clever trick to fool an attacker. Nearby was a rocky wall, and I was sure a moray eel might poke its green, smiling face out from a crevice as I had seen in so many underwater photos. I wanted to see its toothy trickster grin, the long, needle-like teeth.

I spent hours marveling over algae and reef fish, and when the sun was low in the sky, I sat on the rocks, pulling off my mask and fins. As I walked up the beach, gear in hand, the thick, heavy cloak of hypervigilance enshrouded me again.

What had captivated me most though that summer was Sidra. From the marine lab where we worked, Kurt, a senior tech that I had become interested in, brought me over to meet her at the Seaquarium by slipping through a break in the fence between the two properties. I always felt I was sneaking in—a familiar theme in my life—even though the two facilities shared joint research projects, and it was understood that employees could go back and forth. I remember passing the manatees. Heads of cabbage floated atop the water in their tanks. I marveled over the fact that these "sea mermaids" were vegetarian and grew so huge on a diet of leaves.

Sidra was a beautiful gray, white, and pink dolphin. She was sleek and smooth, her skin watery and slippery. Her forehead was streaked with white stripes that converged into a single point in the middle of her forehead. Her body was tapered and streamlined, darting around the pool so fast that I was afraid to get in the water with her. Dolphins are capable of killing sharks many times their size by broadsiding them at high speed with their noses.

Sidra wouldn't hurt anyone on purpose despite her razor sharp teeth. When I hand-fed her, she patiently waited for me to release each morsel. Kurt taught me to pull my hand away from her mouth as soon as I dropped the fish into it, so she would not rip my hand open as she whipped her head away and sped off. When I held the food up over my head, she knew I meant to toss it; she raced across the pool, and as soon as I pulled my hand back, she rose onto her tail, her body hovering miraculously above the surface of the water. I threw the fish over her head, and she leaped to snatch it. She'd fall backwards into the water with a huge splash, dart at high speed around and around the walls of the tank, and pop up in the middle of the pool ready for the next morsel. I loved this game—her dark eyes sparking in sunlight; the shine of her smooth skin; the wonder of her speed. She clicked wildly and every time I'd flip my wrist in a mock throw, her head snapped back anticipating where the food would land.

What touched me the most was how Sidra greeted me. She was dependent on people for sustenance, so she was sensitive to our comings and goings. Long before I even got to the ramp alongside her tank, Sidra sensed my approach and sounded her high-pitched *eee-eee-eeee*. By the time I actually saw her, she was halfway out of the water, making a loud clicking sound, her body bobbing joyfully as her powerful tail held her upright. Her dark, timeless eyes penetrated something in me. I felt recognized, seen. She saw into the me beyond my personality—the essence of me, the timeless me—my soul. No person in my life, except for my Uncle Bill, with whom I rarely spent time, had ever greeted me with such presence and pleasure.

I met Kurt at a graduate school staff party. He was muscular and had eyes that sparkled, and he also loved the sea. He joined me sitting on the floor as I petted Sammi, the hostess's silver Russian Blue cat. I learned about his stint as a helicopter technician in the Vietnam War; his divorce; his work at the lab with Dr. Lothar, designing and building gadgets to help him with his deep-sea research. Kurt was thirty-six and I was twenty-one, a big age spread, but his deep dimples and ready smile outweighed the gap. In many ways, he reminded me of my dad—his better half. Kurt had a big heart and enjoyed making things with his hands.

We began to hang out. Each Friday after work, we hit Guarapo's, a grill down the street from the graduate school, and ordered huge salads heaped with turkey and cheese, smothered with blue cheese dressing—sharp and filling. At some point, after several Fridays, eating salad, crunching into garlic bread, drinking red wine, I followed him home in my old Pontiac Seville. We talked on his porch. Inside, we kissed, we made out. He was a good kisser. I felt turned on. But he wanted to go all the way that first night I'd ventured to his home, and this was too far for me. Another night, I was lying with him on his living room floor kissing and again he pressed me. I said no, and he begged me to let him put his penis just a little ways inside me. I felt like a criminal—though not enough to say yes.

I'd only "done it" twice before, with boys I had known for years. The first time wasn't pleasant—my high school friend thought I was experienced and entered me before I was ready. The second time was the exact opposite. His penis was so slim that I hadn't known he had entered when suddenly it was over, for he sat up and began pulling off his rubber before I had a chance to register what happened. Sexual intercourse was, so far, not a satisfying event. Nor was it a casual thing. My body had been broken into early in my life. Penetration was dangerous. I had to feel completely safe unless, of course, I was drunk. There may have been a third time, with my Everglades friend Rory at his place; after three huge White Russians, who knew for sure?

That first night at his home, I pleaded, "Kurt, can you hold out a bit longer?" How could I explain my situation? I couldn't even articulate it to myself. Was I connecting the dots to that early trauma? No. It just seemed too soon to have sex with Kurt. And maybe I just didn't know him well enough yet. When to lower the drawbridge? When to fortify the walls? That's the thing: The early operation confused things. I was overly defended, which complicated my life. Terror—that intruder—still lived inside me calling the shots. Hypervigilance reigned. My life was not my own.

Every day that summer at noon, I fed Sidra, even on the weekends. Her food was actually medicine. Before heading over to the tank on the opposite side of the grounds, I slit the fish and tucked in some pills before tossing the tasty sea fare into her feed pail. She had contracted a liver disease, which Kurt told me was fairly common for dolphins in captivity. In fact, I was issued a special pass for Saturdays and Sundays to get through the tollgate that allowed me onto Sidra's island: Virginia Key. Illness conferred privileged status—familiar territory. Part of why I had felt obliged to help Sidra in the first place was because she was ailing.

Sidra had a soft, white belly, which she often let me stroke. Her mouth was always turned up a bit because that's how dolphins' mouths are; her "smile" always made me laugh. She swam close to where I sat on the diving board at the edge of the tank and whenever I reached out to touch her nose, she pulled it away playfully and dove under, a game of tag whether I wanted to play or not. When she sidled up to my hand nudging for food, I sometimes looked into the blowhole in the top of her head to see how far down I could see. But Sidra always interrupted by shooting out a stream of white spray.

Besides Kurt and me, Sidra had many caretakers, including Kurt's friend Grace, who had tried to kill herself earlier that summer. Kurt took me to meet Grace. I sensed her misfortune was an omen for my own life. White bandages wound tightly around both wrists. I disliked her, I thought, because of her caustic sense of humor and her fat. In reality, I was afraid of her pain. As a teenager, I too had tried to kill myself. I had worn a white bandage around my wrist, but she wasn't hiding hers. Where was her shame? Still, it made us part of some weird sisterhood. In each of us, a part had risen up to strike us down. When might that killer inside me rise up again?

When summer ended, Kurt moved back to his hometown in Greenwich, Connecticut, and I transferred to Barnard College in Manhattan. We continued to date. Once, we visited his friend Bob, who operated the electron microscope at the Museum of Natural History, and his wife, Kari.

They, too, were much older and had been married for several years. I felt out of place eating at their cherry wood dining table and couldn't wait to get back to the dorm with its funky little kitchen and dining nook. That night, Kurt stayed over in my room. He expected that we would finally have sex. Wrong. "I have a terrible headache," I lied.

Angry—furious, really—he crashed his fist down on my desk, threatening to leave and never call me again. I convinced him to stay, but all night I lay awake bombarded by chaotic thoughts: Maybe I just wasn't normal like other girls; maybe I didn't work on some basic level; maybe some switch was turned off inside me. I did not understand how far I'd run from my body and how severe my state of paralysis. I existed as two entities, mind and body, as far apart as Saturn and the milky blue ball of Earth.

The following week, I took the bus to visit Bob at the museum. He had invited me to see the famed microscope—cutting edge technology in the '70s. I looked into the lens at a shell "millions of years old." To my disappointment, I saw only a pitted surface, crowded with craters and crusty cliffs. Why couldn't I see into the cells themselves to the mitochondria and ribosomes? Why wasn't the microscope revealing chromosomes? Our focus remained on the skin of things.

On the Amsterdam Avenue bus, riding back to my dorm, I sensed my relationship with Kurt was over. I could not yet lower the drawbridge and he could no longer be patient.

The last time I spoke with him on the phone, I learned that Sidra died of liver disease. Kurt thought it best since she had gone blind despite the tarp the staff had stretched over the pool to provide respite from the sun. He also told me that Grace had killed herself. Hearing these things, my body locked. Loss was biting at my heels. I felt enormous dread. Did I sense then that I would try to end my life before the year was out?

My first semester at Barnard, I earned all As and a B and felt relieved, even proud of myself. The academic pressure though had been enormous. Spring semester would be even harder what with taking physics and cell biology at Columbia University, our sibling school across the street. At the beginning of the spring semester, I began to see a specialist for jaw pain and headaches. He diagnosed me with TMJ, tempero-mandibular joint dysfunction, a new diagnosis back then. Besides grinding my teeth down and making me a brace, the doctor prescribed Valium to manage the tightness in my jaw, telling me it was just like aspirin.

That summer, clamming with friends in Barnegat Bay, New Jersey, I threw the pills overboard. Kristina, whom I'd met through a friend at Barnard, warned me that Valium was dangerous. She was much older and wiser than me, had graduated from a sister Ivy League college years before, and was studying to be a naturopath. I idolized her. When she saw me take the vial of Valium from my purse after lunch on the boat, she asked to see it and proclaimed it "poison." That was all I had to hear. Over the side with it!

A few weeks later, I fell into a severe depression. I was apartment-sitting my friend's place in the East Village and couldn't get up off the futon. Hour after hour I lay in a fetal position just beneath her front window, listening to life below on Sixth Street. At night, music and laughter poured onto the sidewalk from the Frog Pond Bar and during the day, distant jackhammers and children's screams filled the air. I lay in my pajamas. Why bother to dress? All I thought about was how messed up I was.

How could I have known that I was in withdrawal from Valium? At the time, this drug was not even classified by the pharmaceutical industry as addictive. After weeks of anguish, I tried to take my life.

A sea creature saved me. Hospitalized on a psychiatric ward following my recovery in ICU, I dreamed that I was standing on a high dive alongside my brother. We jumped together. I don't know what happened to him. As for me, all of a sudden the concrete apron of the pool was directly below, no longer filled with water. Instead of crashing fatally onto the hard surface, I metamorphosed into a heart-shaped organism with thick, brown velvety lobes, a Nigricans alga, glinting gold in sea light—the same type of creature that I had fallen in love with snorkeling years ago and snatched for my algae collection.

That morning, sitting on an orange vinyl chair in my hospital room, I made one of the most difficult decisions of my life. The staff had been pressuring me to leave the hospital. None of the options that the social worker had presented, however, seemed right. I closed my eyes and looked inside for the answer. This move in itself was monumental—a step toward learning to trust my own instincts.

My brother had told me about a treatment program, close to where he lived in northern California, that had helped his friend. The brochure was full of colorful pictures of people playing and working together against a backdrop of ripe, green hills. Men and women playing volleyball, sitting in a circle talking, working in the kitchen, rinsing dishes. A group of runners topping a hill, the Pacific Ocean in the distance. The brochure boasted the beauty of its Marin County location and a philosophy that honored the development of one's innate abilities through the practice of self-reliance. On the front page, a quote from the Synanon Philosophy: *A man is relieved and gay when he has put his heart into his work and done his best.* Synanon's basic rules— no smoking, drugs, or alcohol—were a good fit for me. A commitment to daily work and exercise were mandatory. And for those like me who needed help, the program was free! Kristina helped me figure out that relying on money from my family would be toxic for me.

Though Synanon focused mainly on rehabilitating alcoholics and drug addicts, the organization helped anyone who could not make it on the outside. To me, Synanon was a place of hope, a place where self-discovery seemed valued. There, I might discover my inner self. The brochure's words—*an island of sanity*—struck me. The sharks in the waters surrounding me would be held at bay. The intake meeting went well. I decided to attach my holdfast to a rock in the Pacific.

≈≈≈

Over the course of a year, depression loosened its grip. I worked weekdays at various jobs in the community, joined the choir, and ran over a mile a day. I became fit and felt strong, not only physically but also mentally. I had developed daily habits of journaling, drawing, and meditating—practices I started myself. Synanon did not encourage solitary pursuits, but the lack of stimulus from newspapers, radio, and the outside world in general, plus the constant diet of the philosophies of Emerson and the ideas of psychologist Alan Watts, fueled the desire to know oneself. I wanted to go deeper in understanding.

With the help of my brother, I left Synanon when the program got weird. Men were required to get vasectomies for birth control and single women, like myself, were pressured to marry. I was just beginning my life, just starting to come to terms with my breakdown, my suicide attempt, my stint in the psych ward. I was just starting to accept the fact that I was more attracted to women than men. And Synanon was definitely a hetero world. As hard as it was to leave, I took my brother up on his offer to help me move to Oakland. I lived with him in San Anselmo, Marin County and took buses to the East Bay.

Checking out a co-op bulletin board for rentals, I felt excited about living in the Bay Area and found a flat with a woman named Carla who just quit UC Berkeley in order to train for a job repairing Xerox machines. The mention of her pet hermit crabs on her flyer won me over. I found jobs housecleaning for a living, something I'd done a lot of in Synanon, and planned to spend the mornings reading and writing, hoping to understand why depression had dragged me underwater—the source of those rip tides. I took writing classes at the Berkeley Women's Center and found a therapist who took Medi-cal. I was restarting my life, even seeking out relationships with women. It wasn't long, though, before depression claimed me once again.

One night, I felt especially hopeless, lying on my futon in my bedroom. Out the window, the crescent moon was coldly bright, its edges sharp against dark space, and I felt no real connection to anyone. Friends came and went. My therapist and I could not seem to break through to something real. I was estranged from my mother and father; my brother, tired of hearing how I felt, advised me to "chew nails and get tough." He could not understand me. When I was in high school and college, I'd had a goal. But my dream to be a marine biologist had died. How could I go on with no purpose in life? I felt untethered, drifting about in the sea of the world, unable to anchor and create ties of meaning.

journal, 7/9/77

i cover my eyes
and know of a woman running
hair flying out in all directions
skirt flaring
her mouth open
wailing a sound that echoes
her eyes wide
and dark
and deep
she never stops running
never stops running

the anger and pain

so locked in

she fears facing it

having learned so well

to turn it on herself

so it energizes her running

it fuels her

she is burning herself alive

she is a woman setting herself on fire

she eats herself alive

she will not feel herself

only every once in a while

which frightens her even more

and then she runs even faster

more wildly

usually in the dark of night

you can find her

stuffing food into her mouth

burning a diary

daring some man to pop out of the bushes

    so she can burn him to ash

    with her glare

you can find her always in darkness

laughing

drunk with the knowledge

of the extent to which she's internalized

the pain of her family

drunk with the knowledge of her death

wish, of the extent to which she

is an object of pain

she invites pain, she loves pain, she

cannot live without it

and feeds on showing everyone how much pain

    is inside her

she turns the anger, the pain in on herself

i am a woman killing myself

i am a woman killing myself

i can't stop killing myself

i am self-immolating

filled with hate

when me you see me, hate you know

i am a woman hating myself

mommy

daddy

i learned the lessons well

mommy

daddy

is this the way to twist the knife around and

    around?

is this the way?

7/18/77

is it that i can only feel myself

when i have eaten and smoked enough

to feel myself sick?

courage

is part of me
that i will not know now

i want to stay forever in my bed
masturbating
warm under the electric blanket
i want to stay forever masked, split
unknown to myself
i want to walk forever in the night

a flower bud caught by early frost

i see a blind man
and admire his courage
despise my cowardice

what is my life?
tonight
I see failure
a weak woman
unable to cope
to graduate college
to cry out for help
a woman
who won't change
who resists love
who holds her breath tight in her stomach
and her face tense
who holds the tears in her face
   tight

who is hot and will not take off her sweater

where is the listening?

i feel alone, frightened
trapped
in those defenses that keep us all sane, normal,
    apart
i walk in the night
i walk in the night.

7/29/77

i am so afraid
to feel
i am far away
now
fearing aloneness
fearing
the power in me
tonight
there is no future
moment

my nails dirty
cuticles ripped
the inside of my mouth
bitten raw
my shorts

soiled

my breath

shallow

deeper

with the inhalation

of some life

within me

stuck

sucked in

sucked up

I wrote a suicide note to my roommate and left for Land's End, San Francisco on the coast. Razor blade in hand, I intended to slit my wrist. I sat on the sand, drank some wine, and when I felt a little buzz, made some heartless swipes. I just couldn't do it. Cutting was no longer satisfying. Cutting no longer provided relief. I set down the blade and began writing in the sand. The word *help* appeared. I yearned to be free of self-destructive behavior. I drew an image in my journal that came to me: a stick figure, a cube around its middle, with a black circle in the center of the box; I knew that black circle was my stomach holding me prisoner. Other images emerged. I drew each one. I was onto something.

That night, I slept curled in the arms of a cypress tree's roots and returned to my apartment in the morning to find my roommate's friend, Amanda, who'd heard that I was missing, sitting on my front porch. "I had an intuition you'd be back today," she told me. "And here you are!"

Amanda was the first person in my life with whom I spoke deeply about feelings. When we met in a poetry class a few months earlier, disturbing memories were surfacing, and poetry was my outlet. That day that I returned from the beach, a door opened. I entered.

Amanda not only accepted my depression, she embraced it. She herself had felt hopelessness when she was suicidal as a teenager and, I learned, overcame it through therapy. We sat in her room, talking endlessly about everything. Sometimes, speaking of her family, she cried. I had never seen anyone cry with such abandon. At first, Amanda's eyes squinted and tears snaked down the sides of her nose. Then she wailed, her mouth wide open, front teeth hanging in the air, pink gums exposed. Drool sometimes dripped from her palate before she was able to suck it back. And the laughter that followed!

Amanda laughed until she was unable to make any sound, until all she could do was silently howl, her mouth stretched to capacity, the last of her tears squeezing from her eyes, dark eyelashes wet and shiny. I could no longer hold back and began to laugh, too. Then a sharp "hah . . . hah . . . hah" pierced the air, her final cries. Brow clenched, eyes focused inward, she rattled off insights about her family, searing truths that I feared would burn her to a crisp. Then, she shrieked again, laughter squeezing more tears out of her eyes. I wanted to be able to cry like Amanda.

The comic ironies of life! The craziness! Our shoulders shook, and we flung ourselves onto the couch or bed, wherever we were sitting, letting go entirely, beating the floor, kicking the air. "Stop, stop," I pleaded, "my stomach's killing me!" "How did we ever survive such families?" Amanda cried. We shook our heads and blew our noses, amazed that we had made it to this moment.

The night before I met Lee, the woman who would offer me a magic key to unlock the gate of myself, I had a dream. A large dark purple organ, like a placenta, lies on the floor, liquid seeping into bare wood. I observe it from one side of a room. Like a thick dead worm or a fat liver, it's inert. This blob will never live, I think to myself in the dream. I'll have to throw it out or bury it. Repulsed, I approach the slimy mass, but the longer I stare and the nearer I draw, I see that it is pulsing ever so slightly. It's not dead, I realize. I need to save it! As I bend down to pick it up, I feel faint at the thought of how close I came to disposing of it.

I woke up sobbing in the middle of the night. Scared. After calming myself, I lay in the dark for several hours. When the sun came up, I kept the shades drawn. What if I just stayed in bed, the thick burgundy curtains blocking out the light, and never got up? What if I readmitted myself to a psych ward? What if I threw some things in my backpack and just started walking? Put up a tent in the Oakland hills and lived among eucalyptus and live oak? What if, what if . . .

I scared myself with these questions and biked over to the Women's Center, knowing a therapist was on shift. There she was, sitting behind the desk: dark curly hair, freckles, green eyes. Seeing my puffy face, she clicked on the phone machine and ushered me into a side room. She sat on the floor, leaned against the wall and motioned me to sit between her legs, my back to her front so that I faced away from her.

"I want to cry, but I'm afraid my stitches will break." How stupid that sounded, but these were the words that I heard myself say. "See," I said, pulling up my shirt. "I had an operation when I was 26 days old."

"You can cry," Lee said softly. "Don't worry, your stitches won't break. You're safe now."

The torrents broke through the floodgates. I bawled, cries that erupted from my belly. No words, no explanations, no analysis, no apologies. "Lean back," she offered, and I did—for the next four years.

Seining for Truth
1978–1982

In a dark time, the eye begins to see. —Theodore Roethke

I met with Lee O. Johnson, my therapist, once a week for four years. Lee charged on a sliding scale, typical of those days of the '70s Women's Movement in Berkeley, California. During that time, I lived in a one-room "house" with a tarred roof, a bathroom in the attached hall of the apartment building, and a small courtyard just outside my one window. I parked my bicycle chained to a post and each day biked off to my various house-cleaning jobs, which enabled me to pay the $75/month rent.

In that tiny room, I allowed myself big suffering—grief so ancient, so deep— and my sleep's dreams called me to write them down, not to drown, but to guide me, wake me up, lead me to the light inside. There was a corridor in a crystal cave and I followed it—hollowed out a place in myself to burrow, be safe while the storm raged. Pages of my own writing and artwork filled my room and tears, lots of tears, as I held myself and faced my fears: four years of excavation. Four years of learning to feel, learning to trust my body, unlocking the cage I'd lived in for twenty-six years. A time of hope and healing. I was learning to soothe myself.

That room was a place of revelation—a new self was born, still stiff, still scared, yet vulnerable and more free, more open to life's call. I found that embracing one's suffering allows an awakening to beauty, a polishing of the heart's gem, and a cultivating of soil from which to grow.

Following are some pictures, the drawing of which helped save my life. These images arose from the abyss, the cold, dark depths, craving the light of the world. Some were drawn while in therapy, and others emerged before I met Lee when I was on the beach at Land's End, San Francisco, contemplating a botched suicide attempt and traced the word HELP into the sand. A series of images rose up and as I drew them, I saw that my early surgery was somehow still strangling me. That's when I made my way to the Berkeley Women's Center to find the way back home to myself.

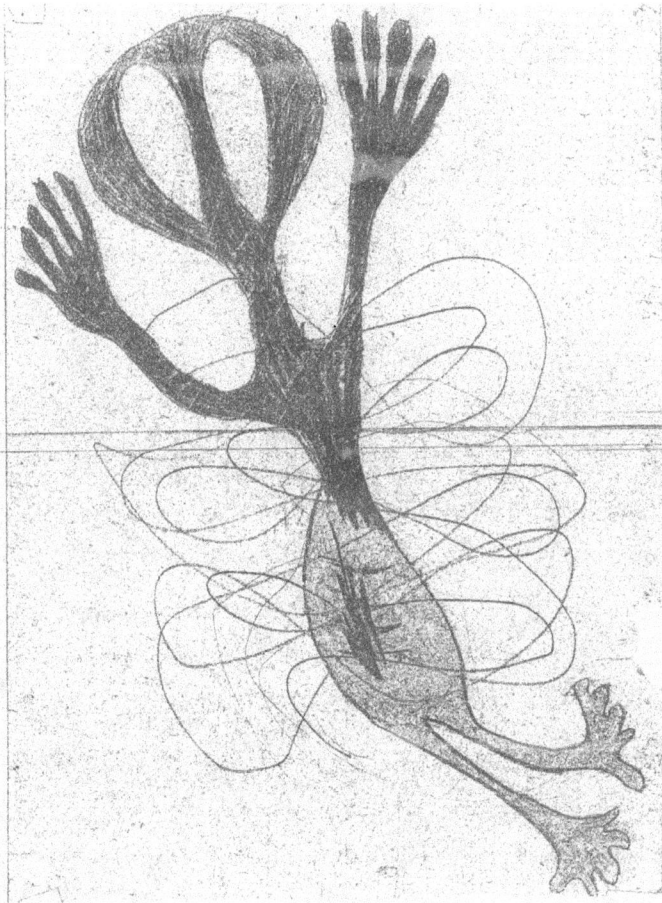

Lee suggested I draw the image I had of myself as a baby. The original drawing was in color: red face, blue belly and legs, and amber eyes on fire.

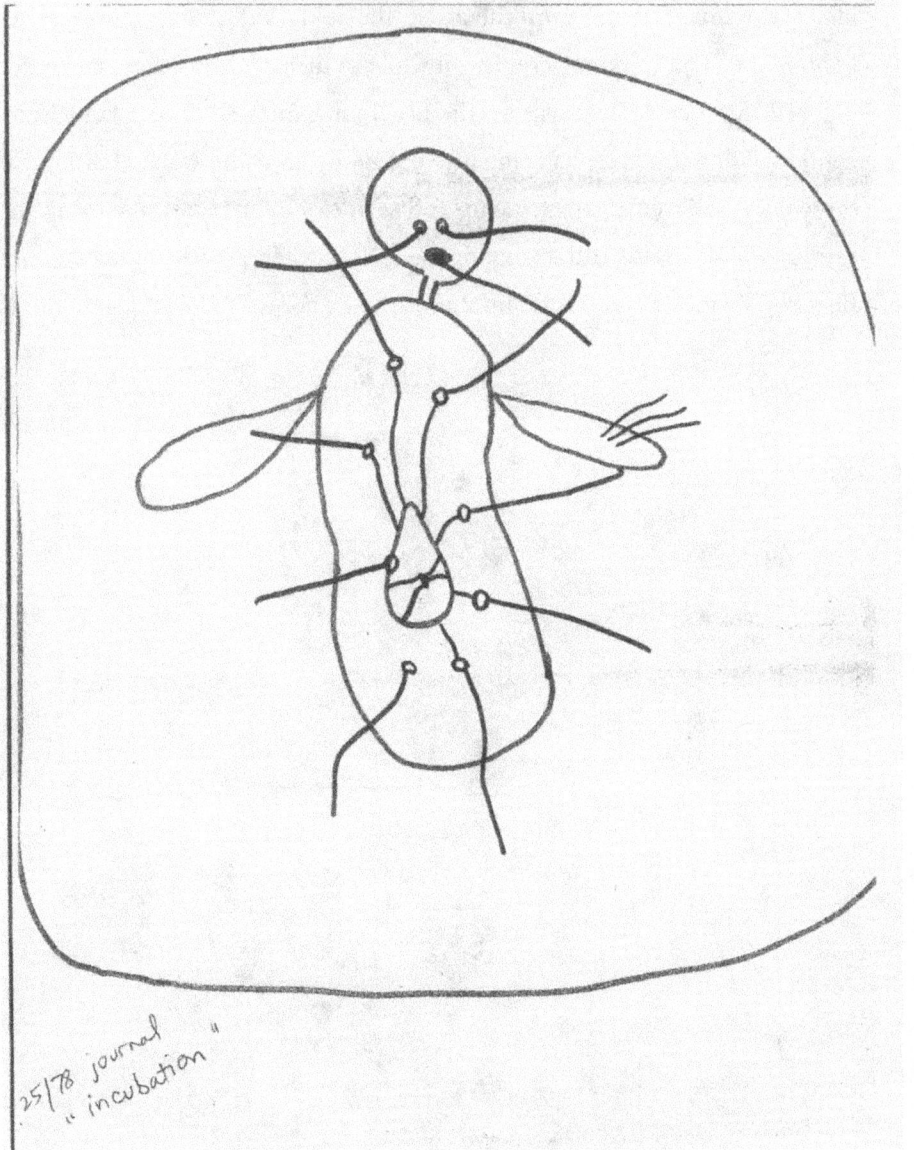

25/78 journal
" incubation "

What I felt I looked like after my stomach surgery at twenty-six days old.

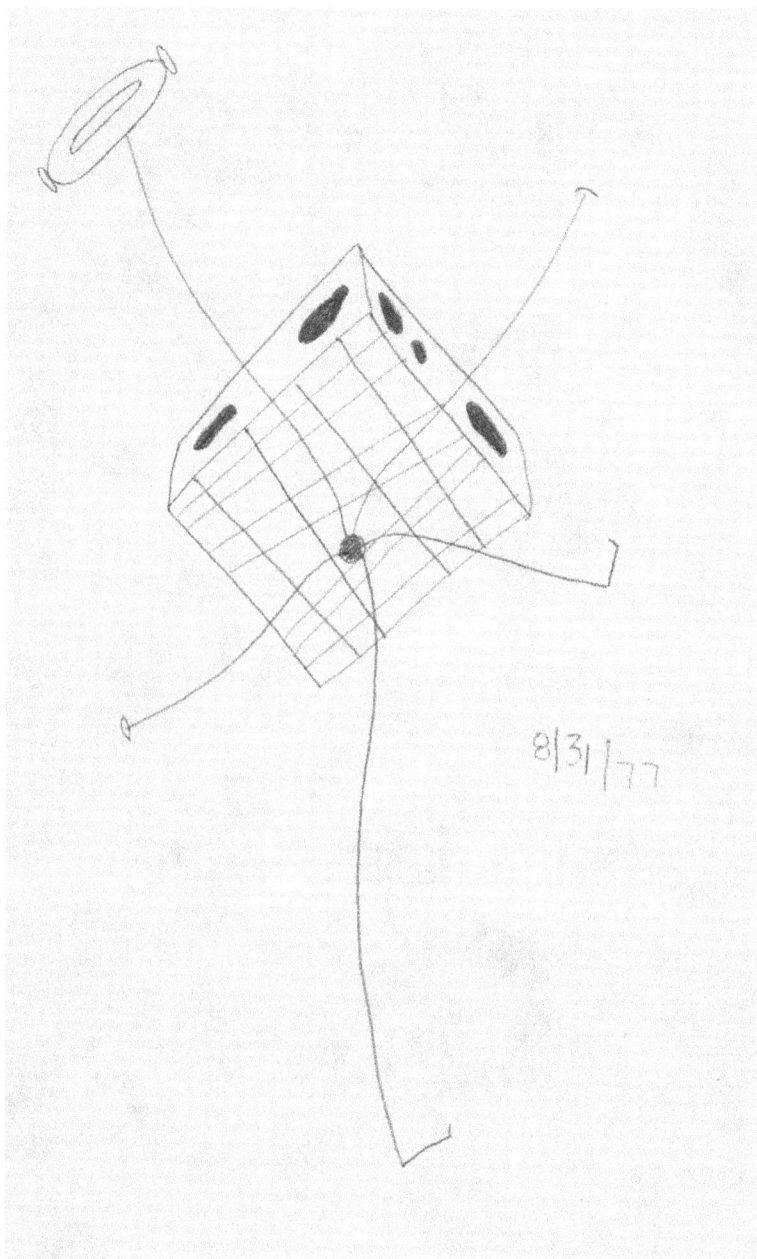

8/31/77

4/15

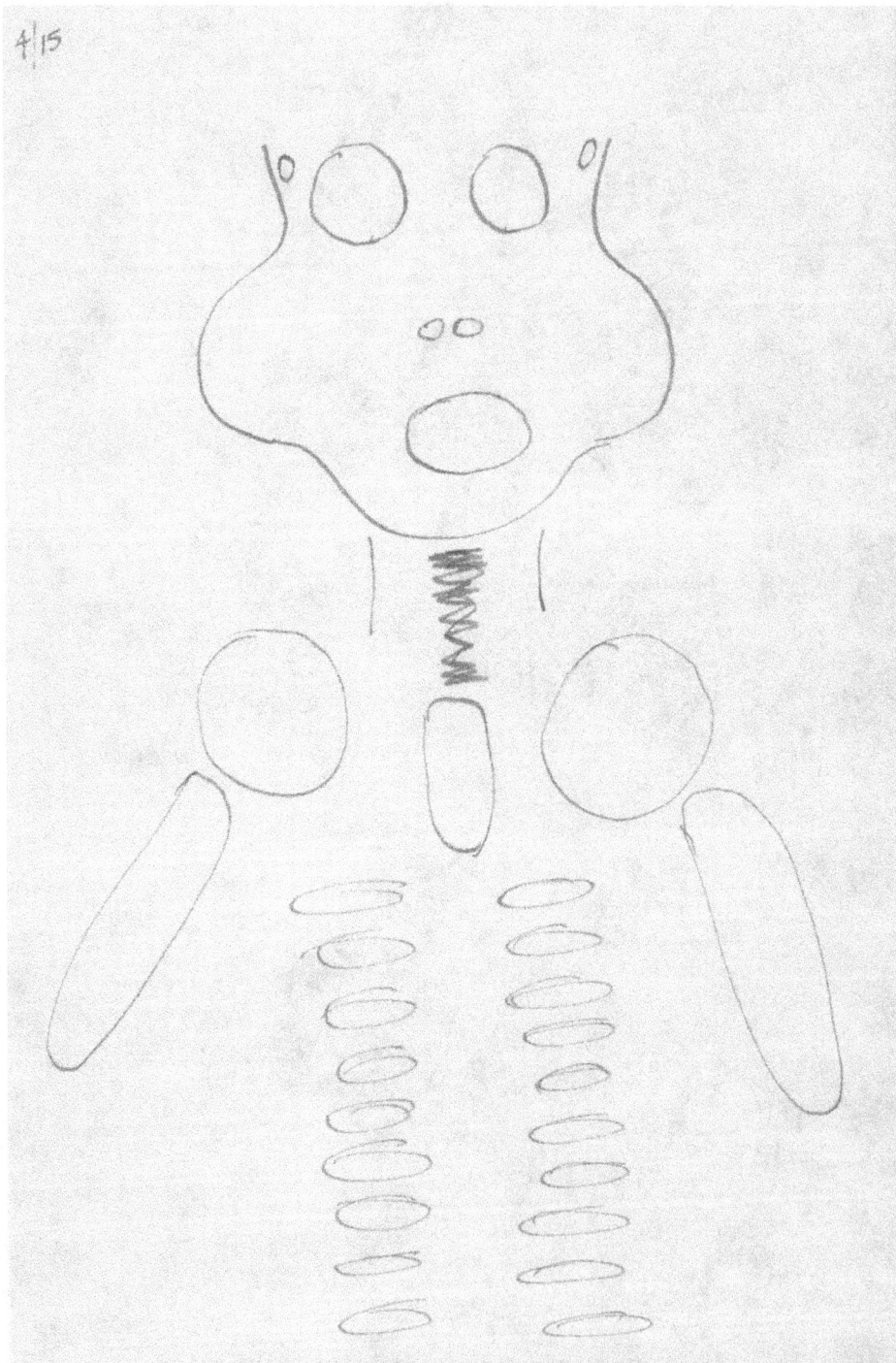

Scream

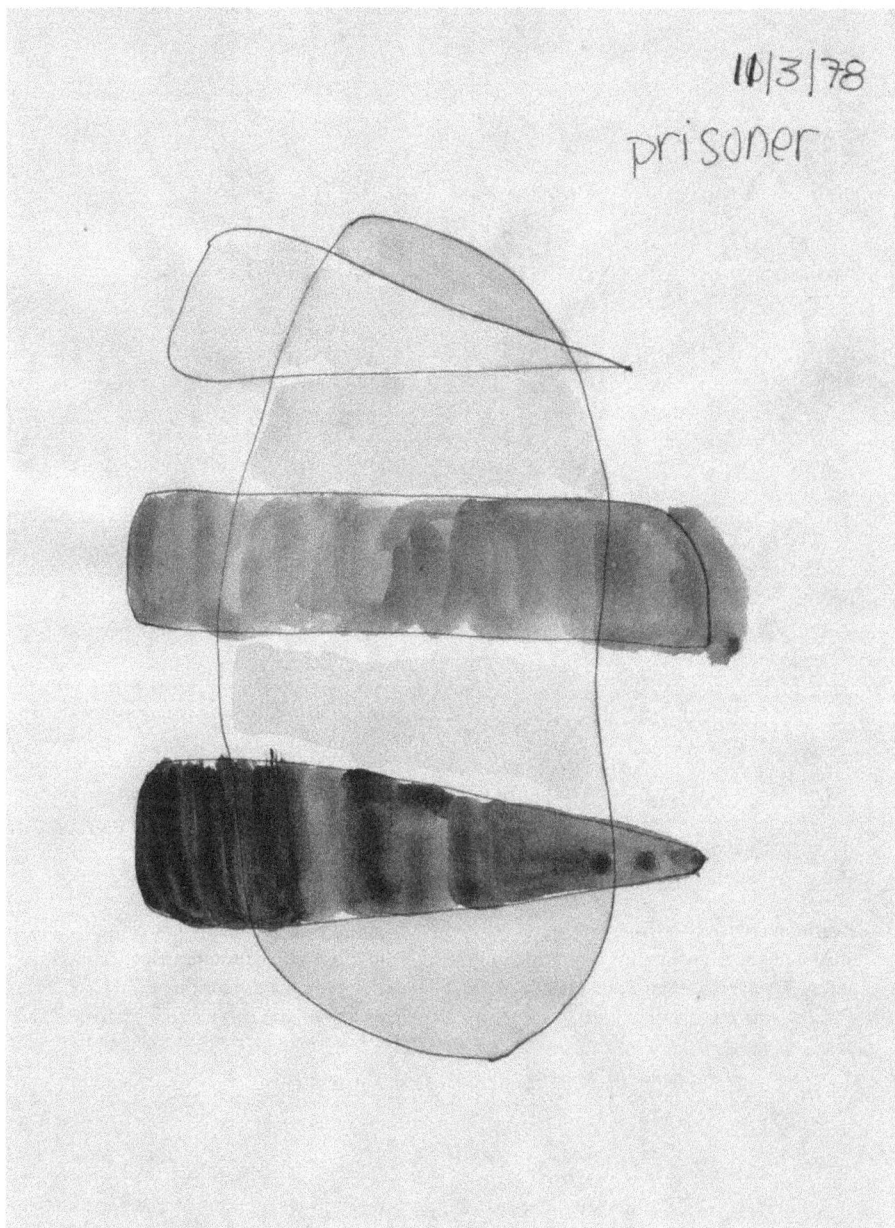

What it felt like to live in my infant-surgeried body for twenty-six years.

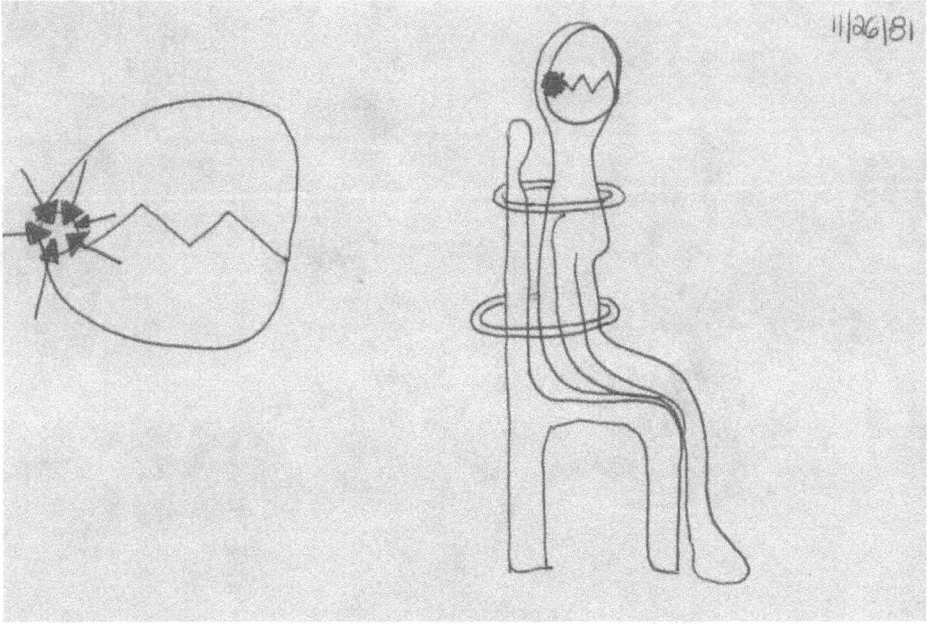

Every morning for as long as I could remember, I would wake up to my jaw clamped shut after a night of gritting and grinding my teeth. On the left side of the drawing, the red arrows point to the jaw pain I felt in my early twenties, which a doctor diagnosed as TMJ or Tempero-mandibular Joint Disorder. Gritting had helped me survive some unbearable pain.

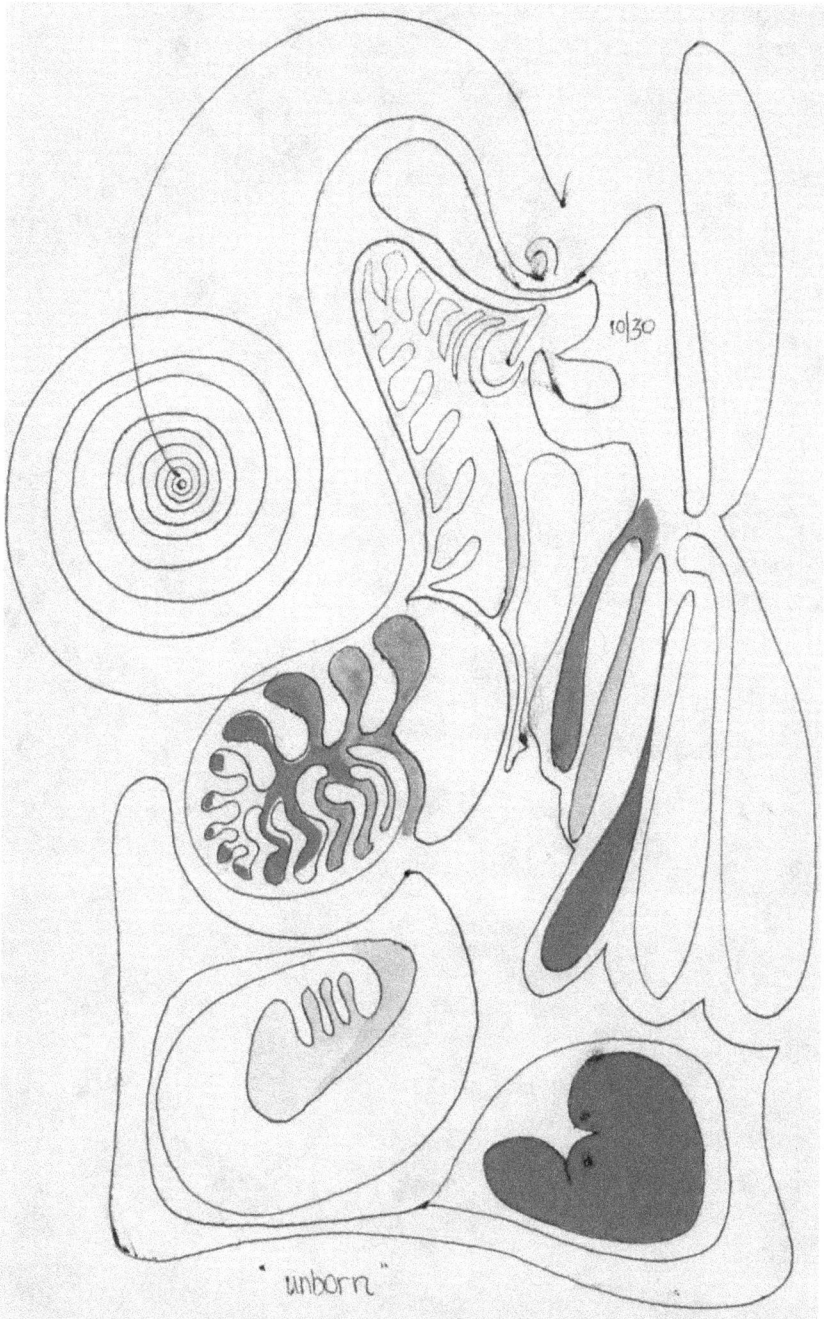

10/30

"unborn"

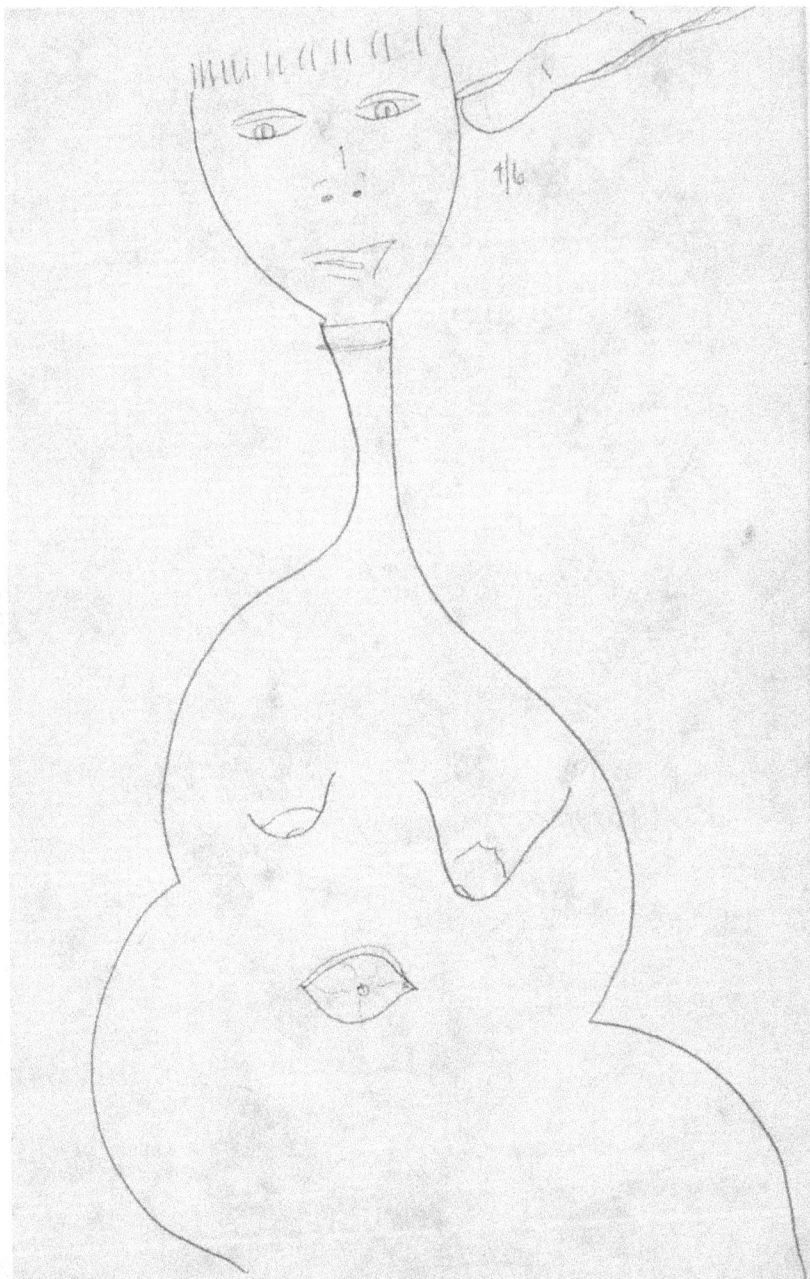

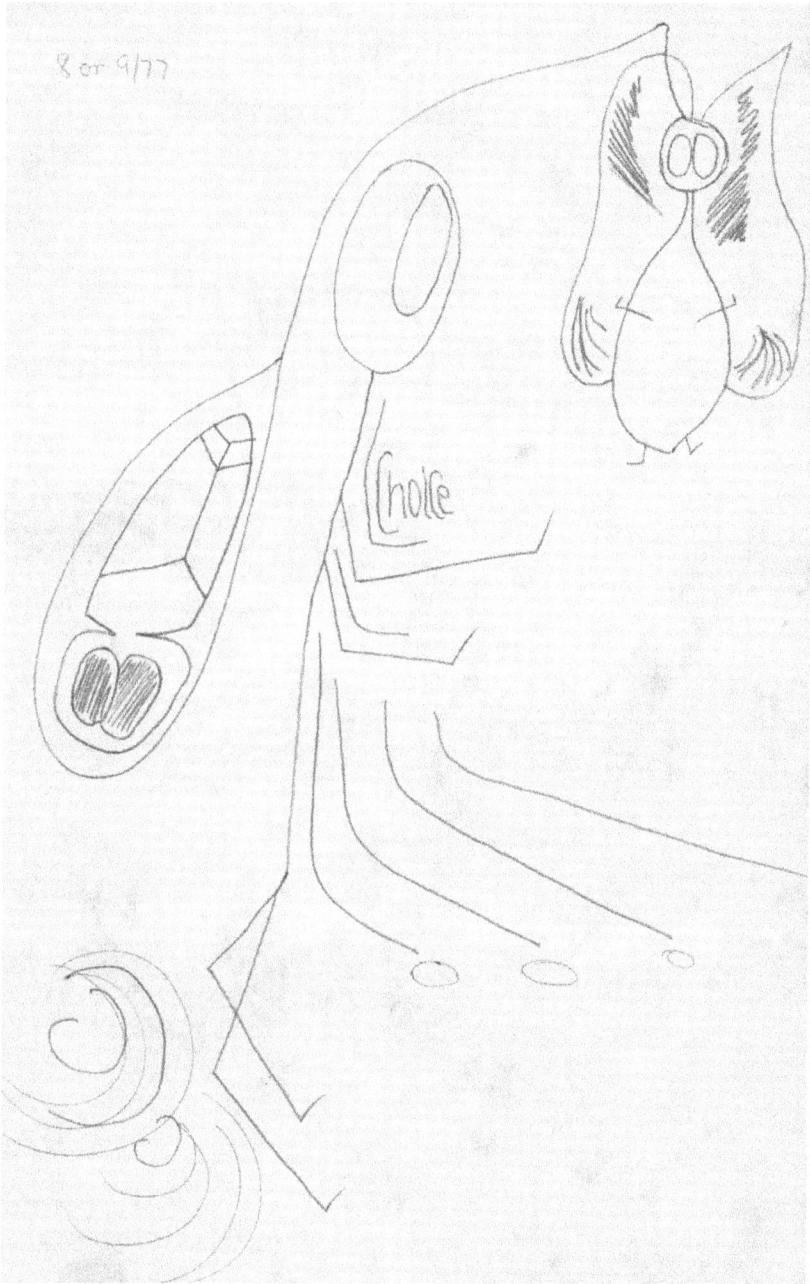

At age twenty-five, I felt unable to move forward in my life. The dead moth of the past was behind me and the butterfly I had hoped to draw in my future was a frozen moth. I was stuck, running in place, and became, once again, suicidal.

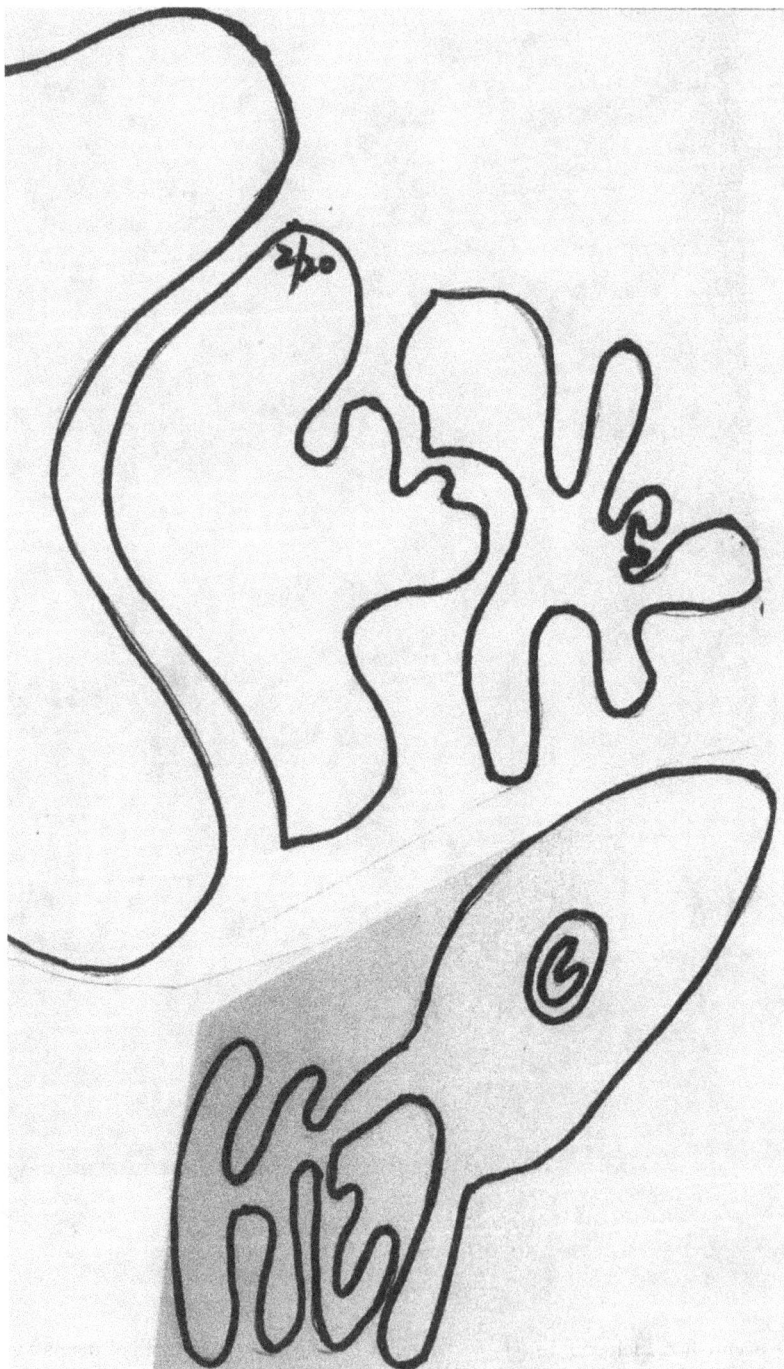

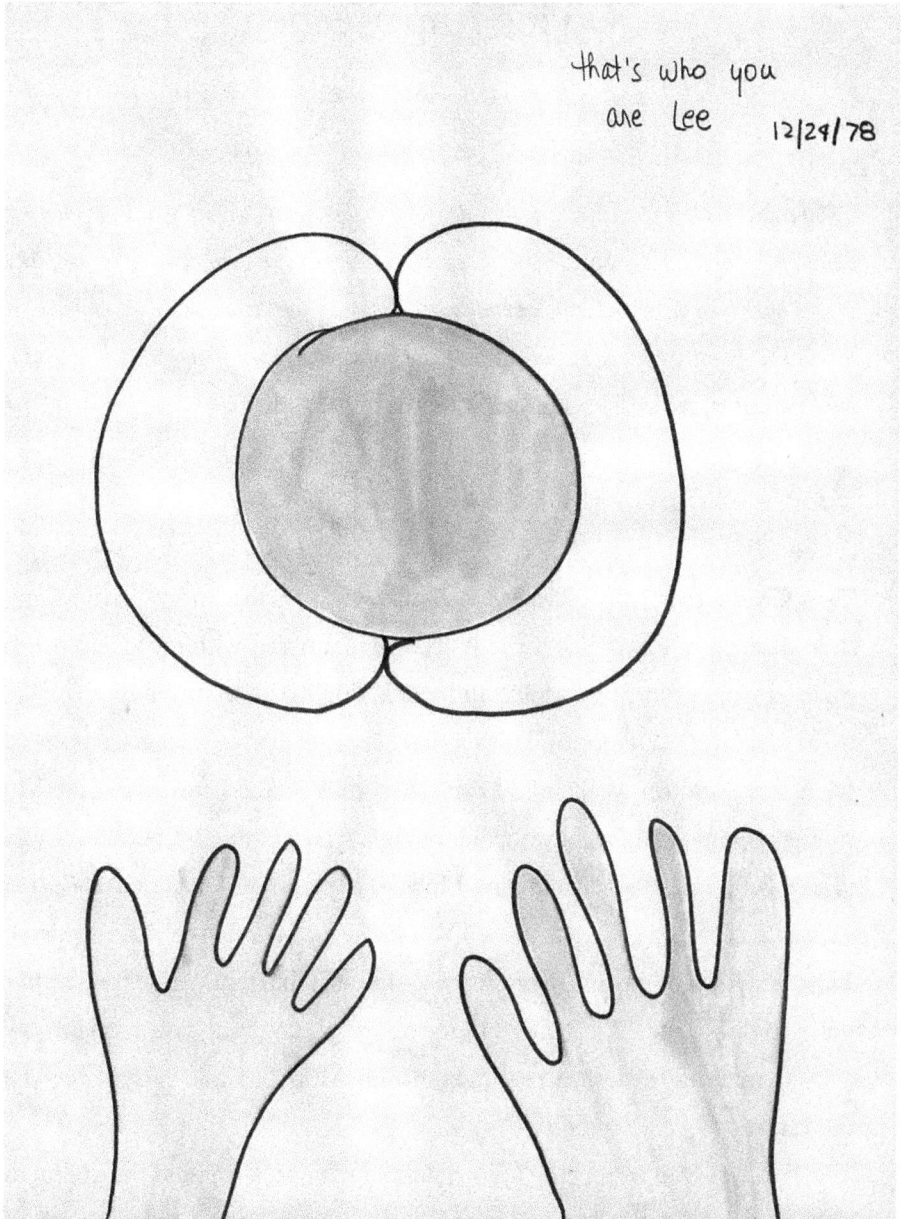

that's who you
are Lee   12/29/78

See me being born? Lee was waiting to catch me as I reemerged from the wounded womb of the past. She was an amazing therapist with a wonderful sense of humor and a skill-set that helped me learn to feel emotions by focusing on what I experienced in my body.

Divine Imperfection

I asked a Hopi woman ... if she selected only the biggest kernels of all one color for planting her blue maize. She snapped back at me, "It is not a good habit to be too picky ... we have been given this corn—small seeds, fat seeds, misshapen seeds, all of them. It would show that we are not thankful for what we have received if we plant just certain ones and not the others." —Dr. Gary Nabhan

My mother calls to wish me happy July 26, the anniversary of my surgery. I have just turned fifty, live in a trailer with my lover Griffin on land in the Sierra Foothills, and teach English at a community college near Oakland, California. During the week, I live in a small studio in Richmond and on weekends, I drive east to the Georgetown Divide. My mother is ninety and still lives alone in New Jersey in the house where I was raised. As usual, she tells me how I looked after surgery—*tubes in and out of every hole, a creature from outer space.* "You looked worse than a dead squirrel. I lost ten years of my life, from forty to fifty just like that." The tone in her voice frightens me. "I'm going to sue you, you know," she says suddenly.

"I must have been a real fighter, huh Mom?" I ask, redirecting the conversation.

"Yes, yes, you were," she admits, taking the cue. "You had the ability to endure. You had a lot of strength that way." This is a first coming from her. Shortly after this conversation, I have an astonishing experience. During an acupuncture treatment, my doctor says, "You have a strong body and a strong spirit." I have never heard anything close to this in my life from anyone. Her words strum a deep chord within, and I sense the truth in what she has said. It takes reaching fifty to consider that this could be true.

I am writing about my operation and feel drawn to it like never before. I am excavating an old sea cave, venturing into my scar, a dark place, seaweed city. In my forties, I had gone back into therapy to talk about it, but we never did break through. The surgery is somehow still holding me back in my life, and I have to find out how. I call Beth Israel Hospital in Newark, New Jersey, where I was operated on as an infant in 1952, but my records no longer exist.

While it's true that I don't remember my surgery, my body does. Perhaps breath memory is a better way to put it. My breath—the way I breathed—changed, probably even before the surgery. The blockage in my abdomen must have been very painful. In any case, I learned to breathe shallowly, above the area that was operated on.

Griffin had been studying Middendorf Breathwork at the Breath Institute in San Francisco for over a year when she suggested I work with Juerg, her teacher. He conducted trainings in teaching breathwork, taught breath classes to the public, and worked one-on-one or hands-on with clients on a massage table, which is how I began.

In order for this type of therapy to work, one has to participate with the practitioner. It's not like massage, where it's important to relax and receive. In breathwork, the teacher follows the client's breath, moving her body in ways that allow the breath where it's been denied or cut off. Life is brought to places in the body that were numb or rigid. Perfect for me—someone for whom the body is dangerous. Someone who can "explode" at any moment. Though I'm better, I still tiptoe around my body, abuse it in some ways, or forget about taking care of it.

Working with Juerg, a dance ensues. His steps are in response to mine. Then, he takes the lead and my body follows. And when the dance is over, breath—and therefore life—fills more spaces of my body. Tissues open to the movement of the breath, like water soaking into a riverbed after many years of drought. With Juerg's hands-on work and his introductory class that I take, I begin to hear the story my body has to tell.

In my first hands-on session, I lie on the bodywork table in the warmth of the round heat lamp, glowing orange. The walls are soft beige and prints of abstract art—few colors but images with long, clean lines—surround. Juerg watches me breathe as I lie on the massage table. He observes where breath moves my body and where it doesn't. "I'm always holding my breath above my scar," I tell him. Juerg says that my breath patterns make sense because when a person breathes, the diaphragm moves the abdominal cavity. I would have experienced pressure, he explains, and after the surgery, this would have caused pain. Also, he says that this running away, so to speak, of the breath is a survival response. "You wanted to save yourself. If you see a cinder block falling that will likely hit your head, you jump out of the way." My breath jumped away from my abdomen and never returned. He slides his large, warm palms under the middle of my back. Breath moves my abdomen, a soft mound that gently rises and falls. The hum of the heat lamp soothes me.

Early on in this process, I happen to see a photo in the newspaper. Surgeons in blue caps and gowns and white masks surround the pink globe of a uterus pulled to the outside of a woman's body. One doctor grasps it with his gloved hands, staring intensely into it as if studying a crystal ball in which the future of the world swirls. According to the caption, he is determining the position of a 32-week-old fetus in order to correct surgically—in utero—a life-threatening condition, resulting from a missing diaphragm. What is the baby going through, I wonder. Has the fetus been given anesthesia? How will this affect her life? Maybe the parents and surgeons believe, as did my mother, that a baby will not feel or remember an operation, that the experience will be a void, a blank space.

I often find a reason for not going to breath class. Griffin, though an intermediate student, insists on accompanying me to the beginner's classes. She knows that I may not go otherwise. She ought to know; we have been together for two decades. In class, we sit on stools in a wide circle. The room is spacious and the ceiling high. Skylights fill the room with light, the glass panes of which are held open by metal rods, lending a vulnerable feeling to the space. To begin, Juerg asks everyone to sit quietly and feel breath movement. "Where in your body do you feel the breath move you?" Juerg then waits for each of us to report our findings. *I don't have a body*, is my usual response, but I can't say that out loud. I settle down a bit and typically realize that I'm holding my breath. *It's ok to breathe now. You won't die*, I tell myself. Breath begins to flow more deeply. I feel breath movement in my chest, but none in my abdomen. It's as if there's a metal pole of rebar wrapped around my middle just under my breasts. *If the breath goes there, I'll die*. Thank God no one can hear me thinking.

"I feel breath flowing nicely in my upper back," one woman says. "I feel breath in my knees," says another. "I feel breath movement in the backs of my shins." What are they talking about, I wonder, annoyed. My turn: "I feel breath in my upper chest. I don't feel my abdomen at all." Juerg nods and smiles a knowing little smile.

I am beginning to listen more deeply for what my body has to tell me. It's not that I've never heeded my body's signs before. It's just that I am no longer waiting for the eleventh hour to respond. I have become interested.

Lying in bed at night, I am afraid to relax. I let myself be carried—a breath term that means allowing my body to know that the earth is supporting me and I can let go—and become alert to signals. I begin to sense breath lifting my chest and moving into my arms and my hands. But I feel afraid of my body. It has failed me before. Who's to say it won't again? I hear the words Juerg uses to ease me into sensing breath movement in my body. *Snuggle in if you can.* A message wells up from deep inside my body— *live to sense and sense to live and don't ever leave me again.*

On the note on the Breath Center door, Juerg apologizes for not being able to let people know beforehand that the evening's breath class is canceled. I feel relief. This feeling is ever so subtle. The thought that followed relief went something like *now I don't have to be in my body. I don't have to deal with not being in it.*

As I lean into my car to get my jacket, I feel myself holding back, leaning onto my heels, not allowing my weight to fall onto the balls of my feet. I am afraid my body cannot support me, I realize.

In sports, when the crucial moment came, I lacked the confidence to deliver. This ineffectiveness troubled me. I was serious about basketball and volleyball and wanted to do well on my high school teams. In basketball, I dribbled into the key and hook shot the lay-up, but the ball bounced off the rim. During practice, I easily made this move. During a volleyball game, when I needed to serve with power, getting the ball as close to the net as possible, no delivery even though I'd practiced perfect serves over and over. Finally, I understand. When the heat is on to perform, I withdraw, fearing my body cannot be counted on to give what is needed.

The other day as I tried to find something while on my hands and knees under my desk, I noticed that I was holding my breath and pulling my stomach in tight. What is this about, I asked myself. *I'm afraid my guts might spill out onto the rug.* It was as if my scar were a zipper that could not be trusted to hold. Of course, I knew this couldn't happen, but my body wasn't convinced. If I breathed fully into the place where the scar was, my intestines might empty like sausage, link after link curling into a snaky pile.

My body has an entirely different way of seeing things than my mind. My cells are awakening, and I am hungry for their stories.

A glare shines into the Breath Center through the glass cubes that make a Z pattern in the white cinderblock walls. We are doing partner work in breath class in which one person faces the other, and have placed, as directed, our hands, one atop the other, over what is called the middle space just below our sternums. For me, this is the place where the scar is. We are taking turns, observing one another from a place of breath awareness as we gently lower and rise in rhythm with our breath. Back and forth we move like a slow seesaw. It is very intimate. While she watches me, I allow my breath into the place that for me is a danger zone. She does not know about my operation and my difficult relationship with my body but goes about her business, hands on her center, lowering her torso and rising. Back and forth, we dance. Perhaps these movements seem ordinary to my partner or to anyone watching, but for me, the experience is profound. I am sharing my operation, in a sense, allowing myself to be observed as I draw breath into that surgeried space of my body. Trust is making its way into my life.

A baby wrapped in thick black tubes, like snakes writhing around her body, appears in my meditation one day. She is alone and could use a hug, yet her face is amazingly serene, except for a slight clench in her brow between her eyes. I pick her up, tubes and all, feel her weight, and smooth her forehead with my finger. I have never held this baby before. It feels so right. *Help me not let her go, I pray. Help me hold onto her for the rest of my life.*

After a meditation group, Linda, a pediatric nurse, told us about an article that she was reading. A study revealed that the single factor that the patients in a psychiatric institution had in common was that they all had been hospitalized in critical care as infants. I knew immediately that these findings were central to my life.

The following week, I visited the preemie ward with Linda. I felt like an honored guest, the graduate of an elite institution. At the nurses' station, Linda introduced me to the staff as a friend who had had an operation as an infant, a pre-op who had only weighed four pounds. The head nurse was thrilled. "Wow, a success story! We never know what's going to become of these little ones."

Before entering the ward, I imagined the babies close to death—tubed atrocities with huge, insect eyes. But as we crossed over the threshold, there they were—adorable little melons, orange cantaloupes ripening in their incubators. I could even see the tiny hairs on their backs. Some were undergoing phototherapy to balance bilirubin, an intense light shining on their chests. Others were barely visible for all the technology, a white ribbed ventilator tube completely covering one baby's mouth and nose. But for all his tubes and the beeping of the oxygen monitor, this baby was human. He pooped. The nurse changed the diaper, and then he pooped again. "Baby!" the nurse said in loving exasperation, "Oh baby!" These beings, gracefully waving their tiny, paper-thin hands in their miniature space ships, were very alive.

When I walked into a larger room, I was amazed to see a rocking chair next to each incubator. At one point, a grandmother, mother, and her three children arrived for a visit. Extra chairs were brought over. I watched jealously as the mother unlatched the small circular door of the incubator and slipped her finger into the baby's palm, which immediately grasped the warm offering. I thought about the fact that I was separated from my mother before the surgery and then for weeks afterward alone in a hospital room, except for the routine visits of the nurses caring for me. Did they touch me with tenderness? I have the impression that I was an ugly baby then, emaciated, skeletal. *Pre-historic, primordial.* Was I repulsive to the nurses? My mother told me that even if she could have held me when I was brought back from surgery, she was afraid. *All those tubes in and out of every opening.*

One of the babies in the preemie ward was a two-pounder and so thin, I could see the flatness of bone beneath the skin of her arm and the length of bone in her thigh. She was curled like a fetus in the womb as if she knew where she belonged and how to stay warm.

A four-pound boy held my interest most. I weighed almost as much just before I was operated on. Had I looked like him? His face was cute, that of a human and not an ancient moth. Through his miniature nose and mouth, he sucked in all the air that he could, his belly pumping hard in and out, a pliant pouch. He wanted so much to live.

~~~

In the years since my father died, my mother and I have become closer. I visit twice a year, summer and Christmastime. I help her with chores she can't manage alone, and we make our ritual visits to different relatives. She's even come out to California several times, the most momentous visit when she attended my graduation from college; I was forty years old and she was eighty. We've softened toward each other, but something still remains of that separation. Every once in a while, we hit a snag; sometimes, this difficulty inched us closer to real communication, but just as often, we run to our separate corners. Then, we fall back into patterns of relating that shield us from bruises. We both wear armor—hers is made of keratin, like a bird's bill; mine calcium carbonate, like the shell of a clam.

Early one morning, I receive a call from my mother's neighbor, Margaret. My mother, she tells me, was taken by ambulance to the hospital. A week or so prior, she had fallen while chopping ice on the driveway. The X-rays had found no break, but she is in so much pain, it seems likely she has an undetected fracture. I book a flight.

Margaret and I visit my mother at the hospital. She is glad to see us but very disoriented. I figure it might be the medication. After two hours of listening to my mother, breaking in with questions and insisting on answers, we finally put the story together. The previous night, disoriented and angry about the fact that the nurse inserted a Foley tube into her urethra, she pulled it out. Then, she got up, walked down the hall carrying the Foley bag, and told the night staff what she had done, holding up the bag. How sad that she had been all alone with no one to advocate for her.

It seemed that the nurse put a restraining jacket on her and locked her into what my mother called a "high chair," a seat from which she could not get free. According to my mother, she sat there for four hours, cursing out the nurses. Margaret and I are shocked.

I find the charge nurse and tell her to please call me if my mother becomes agitated. I will come right to the hospital—no restraints! She notes this on Mom's chart.

"I'm going to write a letter when I get out of here," my mother says as I'm leaving. "I'm going to blast them on the front page of the *Elizabeth Journal*."

For the first time in the almost two weeks since my mother was hospitalized, she sits in a chair next to her bed. The CAT scan shows that she fractured her lumbar spine in two places. She's been transferred to the geriatric ward for physical rehabilitation at a different campus of the hospital. With rest, physical therapy and progressive ambulating, the doctors feel certain she will be able to walk again. I sit across from her on a brown Naugahyde chair.

She talks about my babyhood—that I had a wonderful appetite. She says that I wanted to eat everything. I ate whatever she put in front of me and was happy. "You were the kind of baby who wanted to get up and go.

You had pep. You didn't want to wait for anything." She grabs onto the arms of the chair and pretends to push off, her eyes wide. "'*Let's go already. What's next?*' you always seemed to be asking. You weren't content with just sitting around."

I am floored. She has always led me to believe that I was a lump of a baby, immobile and docile—*wrapped up in all those tubes!* A sack of rocks weighing her down. Burden baby.

"After your problem, you were just great."

I feel furious. Why didn't you tell me this before, I want to yell. If I had heard this as a child, I would have lived an entirely different life! Had she shared positive messages, but I just never was able to hear them? No. It was all about her trauma. I want to scream at her, but where will this type of response get me, I think.

I remember a baby photo of me taken long after the operation—me sitting in my jump seat, my mouth wide with joy. I was eight months old. That's the baby my mother was talking about. "Sun baby," my friend called me upon seeing that photo. I was *that* baby. But Mom rarely spoke about her.

The morning before my flight back home to California, I visit my mother at the rehab hospital. She is lying on her side. "I have a pain in my hip that I haven't had before," she tells me. "And when I walk, I hear a clicking sound."

Her physical therapist says that it makes sense. "Your mother did a lot of walking this morning and without the walker. We made it all the way down the hall and back. Now, her hip needs a rest."

After reassuring my mother the pain is to be expected, I try teaching her a lesson in body awareness. "Mom, there are ears all over your body. You've got to start talking nicely to your hip. It hears everything you say."

"Yes, I've been telling it that we've got to get out of here."

"How did it respond?"

"*You're telling me, toots*, it said."

A month after she had been taken away by ambulance, my mother is finally home from the hospital. Her spine is healing well, but she moves more slowly and on some days, uses two canes to get around. I fly back to see her again a few weeks later. Before bed, she shows me an injury on her leg. It's a serious cut, deep and red, almost the size of a dime, the skin purple all around it. On closer inspection, the wound looks like pizza, puffed up cheese and tomato sauce. Referring to it, she pokes her finger right in.

"Mom, you're sticking your finger into it!" After pulling her finger away, she goes on talking about the wound and jabs her fingertip in once more.

"Mom, you did it again. You're going to infect it!"

She scrapes the surface as she points to it, trying to understand what she did wrong. I literally swat her hand away. I feel anxious. Lately, her skin has not been healing well. In fact, on the back of her hand is a large red wound without a scab, still raw from an injury she sustained over a year ago. Her skin tears like tissue.

"What is this purple spot here?" she asks, brushing the wound once again.

"Lie down, please, Mom." This way she simply won't be able to reach the cut, so I can wash it in peace. Lying on her side, she looks content in her flannel nightgown, a pattern of yellow lilies against a blue sky, her arms still at her sides. A rare moment.

I press a warm washcloth over the wound.

"Ooooh," my mother says, "that feels nice."

I clean out the fatty stuff, swipe on antibiotic cream, and bandage it.

"Mom, look at your skin. It's so dry. You should rub cream on it every night." Her heels and lower legs are covered with a light, white netting that looked like spider webs. "The skin is flaking."

"Nothing you can do about it, Wend. It's just what happens when you get old."

"Yeah, but you could take care of it by putting cream on every night." I rub lotion over her feet and lower legs. I often give good advice about how others should take care of *their* bodies, I note.

"Wash your hands good when you're finished there, Wend. You might pick up something. Remember Aunt Mable and her purple feet?"

As I turn to go to the bathroom, I notice my high school graduation photo on the shelf above the sewing machine. My face is expressionless—almond-shaped eyes encased in black eyeliner; straightened hair; bangs pulled flat to one side; lips pressed together. "There's dead girl," I say, pointing to my photo.

"That's my favorite picture of you," my mother defended. "I don't know why you call it that."

My mother's mind is disintegrating. At one o'clock in the morning, she bursts into my room, claiming that I was chasing her. "You chased me over the bed and all around the house and wouldn't stop." She pokes my thigh accusatorily. "I came in here to see if it was true. I can't believe you're in here under the covers. You were chasing me." She pokes my thigh again, this time harder.

"Mom, I've been right here all night," I say, upset, afraid of her. Even though she's ninety, my mother is still very strong.

"But you were chasing me. You wouldn't quit. You were everywhere, even climbing over my bed." She acts as if the experience is still happening.

"I haven't left my bed," I argue. She continues to stand beside my bed, leaning toward me with her hands slightly raised, as if ready to defend herself. I am prepared to grab her wrists if I have to. "Mom, go to bed. I have a plane to catch tomorrow. It's late. You had a bad dream."

"I don't know. You were chasing me. Why wouldn't you stop?" I lie back down and pull up the covers. Reluctantly, she turns and leaves.

In the weeks since I've arrived home, my mother has begun walking without a cane, taking care of the house, paying her bills and unfortunately, driving. I'm worried about her and phone often. During one call I mention that I have a birthday coming up, number 52, then wish I hadn't as I anticipate her response.

"No," she says, "you have two birthdays. That was such a suffocating time. I would much rather not remember. In fact, I don't know how I ever got through it."

"But it was a good time, too, wasn't it? I survived."

"Yes, it was, but you know, I'll probably remember that surgery after I'm dead."

∾∾∾

While doing a spinal roll in breath class, lowering vertebra by vertebra – a sort of slow motion touch-your-toes exercise – I feel frightened my spine will not support me. In bringing breath awareness to my neck and back, I find that as I approach the area behind the scar on my abdomen, I hold my breath. This is uncomfortable. I am not able to continue folding over while holding my breath. In a way, my whole midsection is frozen.

Using the Principles of Breath, I allow myself to be carried, a term meaning supported by the floor and hence, the earth, and lean into those vertebrae, trusting they will hold me. As I stretch downward, breath flows into that area of my spine, and I complete the exercise without pain. Slowly breath work is doing its magic. Little by little, sensation returns to the places I abandoned so long ago.

≈≈≈

You drive alone to the University of California at Davis, feeling fortunate there's a medical library dedicated largely to historical texts just an hour from where you live in the foothills. You pull into the huge parking lot, insert however many quarters into the meter to ensure an eight-hour day, and push the glass door open, noting how empty this library is. How few seem to want to know its secrets.

The woman at the front desk directs you downstairs, down to the historical material, down to the stacks at the back of the large room, down to the copiers and computers. As you descend, you see the earnest young men and women—doctors in training—backs hunched at the computers, hands on mice scrolling and searching. But you are no young doctor wannabe.

It's because of your body that you are here. You have been so rigid and frightened all your life long. You want to know the story of the scar on your belly. At fifty, you are ready to write your own version of what happened with the stomach blockage you suffered as a twenty-six-day-old baby. You won't die of pyloric stenosis or even be affected adversely by it again. Ridiculous to be afraid? Yes. But not to your body.

You read the Chamberlain article and learned that most infants in the United States before the 1980s weren't given anesthesia for invasive medical procedures and surgeries. In experiments in 1941, babies were systematically pricked with blunt safety pins: their grimaces, cries, and withdrawal of limbs chalked up to reflexes because, it was believed, infants' nervous systems weren't developed enough to transmit pain impulses.

You learned that sick babies were given a muscle paralyzer to stop them from fighting back. You know about the Lawson parents going public in the '80s about their son's death after a heart artery was tied off without anesthesia. Thanks to Dr. Anand and Dr. Hickey, it was finally established that infants do feel pain and that they can tolerate anesthesia. You were astounded and as you learned these facts, you became determined to know more.

You walk to the back of the room as directed—shelf after shelf of fat books about pediatric surgery. Old books published in the '40s, '50s, and '60s. Books about technique with diagrams and pictures. You feel overwhelmed but make yourself scan the titles: Operative Technic, Doctor Conrad Ramstedt and Pyloromyotomy, Congenital Hypertrophic Stenosis of the Pylorus, An Account of the Dissection of a Child. *You carry the heavy, dusty books to the back desk in the corner, sit on an orange plastic chair, and sneeze opening* Operative Technic, 1955 *to the pyloric stenosis entry.*

You learn that you would have had three sets of stitches, not the two sets that your mother had told you about while making Thanksgiving pies: a stitching of the abdominal muscles, a closing of the abdominal wall, and a stitching of the skin of the belly. Maybe four, given the ones your mother mentioned that the surgeon described to her on the stomach's pylorus itself. You skip to the black and white diagrams and feel queasy, seeing the pictures of each step of the surgery. You hone in on the image of the pylorus part of the stomach pulled outside the abdomen by forceps.

Your legs weaken as you walk to the far desk, the weight of hundreds of rows of thousands of medical tomes depressing your shoulders. The fluorescent light strikes the page. The air inert as in bubble wrap. You feel suspended, adrift, disconnected. You are crying as you write this; feeling alone was part of the wounding. How by-yourself your life has been in many ways.

You plant your feet, draw breath slowly into your washboard belly, and look again at the diagram. The surgeon has pulled the "pyloric tumor" of the stomach and part of the small intestine out of the baby's body. The fears that you felt over the years about your guts spilling out were not irrational fantasies.

You slam the book closed, squeezing your eyes shut to prevent tears, and tell yourself to get a grip. If you stop for every tear, how far will you get in a day? Do you really want to come back here? You can't feel your feelings about this, not here. Not when you have zillions of articles to find on the library computer databases. Not when you have to get change so you can feed dimes into the copier, take a lunch break, and do all this before 4:30 pm. Keep going.

You open Operative Technic *again. There it is—the baby's stomach actually being lifted out its belly. The text states how fortunate it is that the liver holds back the intestines from "extruding" or flopping out. You feel sick and look for the bathroom signs, thinking you might throw up; instead, you put your hand over your belly and breathe into it.*

Another book discusses the preparation of an infant for surgery. You haven't ever thought about this and notice your jaw clenching. Before the operation, babies' stomachs are emptied with a nasogastric tube. How on earth, you wonder, did you at 26 days old deal with its insertion? You remember the ICU after your suicide attempt—the difficulty you had with the tube inserted into your nostril, down your throat, and into your stomach. Gagging as the doctor inserted it, you told yourself that it was the tiniest of straws and there was plenty of room left in your windpipe to breathe. You imagined a cavernous sewer with a thin pipe running along the inside. Your imagination and reasoning saved you. But as an infant?

One chapter shows photos of actual babies with their eyes blackened out to prevent identification, ghoulish-looking creatures illustrating techniques of intubation, or the insertion of a breathing tube, into an infant's throat. You hadn't given a thought to the idea that you might have been on a respirator during surgery. Your fingertips rest on your neck as you read.

One photo illustrates intubation technique: a nurse holds down the shoulders of a month-old baby onto a gurney while the doctor works a thick instrument into the baby's throat. You recall the picture you drew in therapy years ago of yourself as a baby—blue hands held palms-up as if to say STOP! The image is a record of the trauma.

When you get to the article about the longitudinal incision popular with surgeons in the '60s versus the vertical one, you can hardly stay seated. Surgeons claimed the longitudinal cut was cosmetically better. Sure enough, the photo of this type of scar looks like the thin, pleasant smile of the Mona Lisa. "With this longitudinal cut, surgery time is shorter and fewer nerves and bloods vessels are cut." The stomach is not pulled from the body, for after the initial incision, the pylorus bobs up easily as the skin and muscle are stretched by forceps, and the surgeon cuts while it lies within the confines of the body.

No such luck for you. In 1952, pulling stomachs out of babies' bodies was in. You picture your own scar—that raggedy, jagged set of crossbars that looks like a brand on a cow. You slam the book shut and scrape back your chair, embarrassed for the noise you made in this most respected institution. But damn, your scar is an ugly rip and you can't stand thinking about it.

It's all too much. The cafeteria is just steps away from the library. Time for a break, get something to drink. You'll just have coffee, you think. Who can eat after seeing those images? But the smell of fried foods gets your juices going. You park your briefcase next to your chair, observing at the nearby tables the young students wearing scrubs in gentle blues and greens. A few adults claim the tables against the wall, some in scrubs, some in suits. On the overhead TV, images of fire trucks, red lights flashing off and on, but the set is too far away to hear. You order a tuna melt.

Once upon a time after your marine biologist dream died, you wanted to be a doctor. You worked as a ward clerk on the gynecology and the internal medicine floors. Later you clerked on Labor & Delivery and then trained as a telemetry technician, reading the heart monitor in the ICU, CPU, CCU—intensive care units—and then on the cardiac ward for several years. You remember with disdain the doctor who called you into a patient's room and had you peer into her cavernous bed sore. Oh, the pleasure he got from the look on your face. You remember concluding that perhaps you did not have the stomach for doctoring.

1:30 pm. Get going, girl, you tell yourself, taking a last sip of cappuccino and gathering your materials. This time, no one at the desk smiles at you as you pass. A solitary, solemn affair. You descend again. On the bulletin board, you notice advertisements for a wildlife veterinarian program that you would have been interested in at one time.

Your biggest find that afternoon—the Solnit and Green article about VCS, Vulnerable Child Syndrome, when a child is traumatized by a parent's attitude about a child's earlier surgery or condition. There is the story of a Mary, an eight-year-old girl who had constant headaches, colds, and pains in her stomach, arms, and legs. "Sickly," her mother called her, complaining that her illnesses interfered with school and friendships. When the pediatrician asked about Mary's medical history, the mother teared up, telling how her daughter almost died from diarrhea and convulsions as a toddler, conditions which had completely resolved. The doctor realized that the mother's anxiety was negatively affecting her daughter's health. If a physician recognizes a situation like this early on and makes a VCS diagnosis, a child has a chance for intervention to alleviate problems,

*such as "difficulty with separation, infantile behavior, bodily overconcerns, and school
underachievement." The child has a crack at normalcy.*

*You hear your mother's mantra again: "Tubes in and out of every opening. You were
an alien from outer space!" Leaning back on the metal folding chair, your chest tightens
with rage at her words; at your pediatrician who filled you with worry year after year;
at the grammar school psychologist who pulled you out of class each week to interpret
Rorschach cards, threatening to send you to a convent; at your surgeon whose words "if
she cries, she dies" froze your mother, turning her touch to ice. "Kill, kill, kill, kill, kill,
kill, kill!" you hear—King Lear raging in the thunderstorm. You are a red-hot pot at boil,
spilling over the lip.*

*You stand up, grab your purse, and walk quickly, tracing the periphery of the library,
past shelf after shelf, row after row, the years of medical history piling up—dead babies
tossed down medical waste chutes, traumatized children, like zombies, filling the rows
of books. You pace up and down the aisles, yearning for release. You bound up the steps
out into the green of the quad in front of the library. A slight breeze lifts the branches of
the sugar maple. The sun warms you lying on the bench. Fresh air fills you for the final
assault.*

*You descend, determined to find something, anything about the practice of using curare.
You know it was used to paralyze sick infants before surgery because medicine believed
in 1952 that babies don't feel pain and anesthesia was too dangerous to use on infants.
Instead, you find other important articles:* Effects of starvation in infancy (pyloric
stenosis) on subsequent learning abilities; Effect of Operative Procedures
on the Emotional Life of the Child; Surgical History: The Story of Pyloric
Stenosis. *You dutifully thunk the heavy journal collections down onto the glass of the
copier, feed in dimes, press <C>, and stack the books on a metal cart.*

*You are losing steam. You've been at it all day: breathing dead air, scrolling through
hundreds of call numbers, reading small print abstracts, and taking copious notes. You
give in to weariness. Your lower back hurts. You stack the books back onto the carts, hoist
up the heavy black briefcase filled with evidence, and ascend, waving to the librarian on
the way out. You've seen the photos. You studied the graphs. You noted procedures. You did*

your research.

Driving home on Route 50 though, you reflect on your talk with the librarian after lunch. She asked what your project was and you noticed her eyes widen with shock as you told her. You went numb, outside your body, talking as if you were the puppet of a ventriloquist, a familiar feeling whenever you try to tell someone about your infant surgery. You hoped you sounded professional to the librarian, knowledgeable. You wanted her to believe you. She searched earnestly for an article about the use of the muscle paralyzer curare on infants with pyloric stenosis. She tracked down the call numbers of different journals, and you were relieved that she appeared to take you seriously. But did she secretly think you were crazy?

As you pull into your driveway, tears break through. You pull onto a side road on the property and stop the car. Reality hits: You were tortured as a baby—tied down, a tube shoved down your throat, drugged with a paralytic, and forced to be awake through surgery. You scream, collapsing over the steering wheel, sobbing. Finally, you can let it all out. You are raw, open, the clouds and manzanita your only witnesses.

Your roller-coaster life now makes sense. You aren't crazy. Your life has been a normal response to trauma. You turn off the car and fall onto the seat back, breathing the sweet mountain air. There's still so much to process but for now, you can pause. The sun is casting its final gold on the foothill's red earth. Chunks of white quartz sparkle along the road. The truth of your own story buzzes like bees over blossoms.

≈≈≈

There is a photo taken of me at four months old, the first since the operation. I am sunken into a huge black armchair, which practically absorbs me, a tiny baby in a blousy, white dress with a large, pale bow. My eyes are two shocked black dots. I look haunted.

"You didn't smile until you were three months old," I remember my mother telling me.

"Why not?" I asked.

"Nothing to smile about."

I dream that I am engulfed by a huge spider web and am fighting to get out. Every time I try to disengage my arm, I am more entangled. Frantic, I pull my shirt off though the spider might fall on me. I do whatever I have to do to get out, and if the spider bites me, so be it. I am sweating. The harder I fight, the stronger the web sticks.

Later in the dream, I observe a different web from across a room. It is a wonderfully amazing thing the shape of a bed, higher at one end as though a pillow were there. The strands zigzag every which way like those of a black widow and shimmer like glowing white lace. In the web is an iridescent butterfly—very still, wings spread wide, its colors, brown, white and a touch of green—where my heart would be if I were lying down in the bed.

When I wake up, the message of both dreams is clear. We can fight what has happened to us, or we can admire the beauty of the web that has been created from our difficulties.

Thinking about this, I feel the flow of breath move my belly. Breath moves my tummy, gently lifting it and letting it down. The iron binding below my ribs that cinched my midriff for over fifty years has loosened its grip. Quietly, a major transformation occurred. The prison gates have swung open. A spell has been broken.

Breath is the book of the soul. In a way, it is my earliest recording of self, a code I decipher to learn the story about what happened to me, given that I have no verbal memory of the surgery. I do have breath and body memory. The way that I breathe tells part of the story. The absence of sensation of breath in parts of my body reveals more. Perhaps breath is the most accurate language I have to describe that time as a fossil or a pictograph reveals ancient beginnings of which we have no written account.

Reading the breath is like reading the signals of a heart monitor. The waves deliver messages. Understanding the peaks as well as the troughs in between is essential. This process requires awareness of subtleties. Once one learns the language, results are guaranteed. Breath is reliable. Honest.

I write my mother about a dream I had, copying the words right from my journal: *A photo of my mother, the upper half of her body. She is beaming. She is young, full of happiness—a tearful joy. Her eyes are dark and wet. This photo was taken right after my mother gave birth to me.* I am so happy to have received this dream, I write, because I grew up thinking what a great burden I was to you and our family. The dream helped me, I told her, to see another side.

My mother writes back: "I was amazed at your dream. Don't think I felt you were a burden. That never, ever entered my mind. My only fear was that something was just going to wipe you out and leave me a sad woman all my life."

"I'm embracing my imperfection," I tell Griffin.

She looks at me with a mix of happiness and skepticism. "Really?"

"Really." I have just come home from my writing group. The woman at whose home we met suggested that we choose some pears from her prolific fruit tree to take home. A friend and I paused to consider which to pick. I reached toward one and turning it gently, discovered a brown blemish. I let it go and began to reach for another when I remembered my dream about the butterfly. This scarred pear just might be the juiciest. I pulled it from the branch.

In the book *My Grandfather's Blessings*, author Rachel Naomi Remen writes about the intentional error always made in a stitch on a Persian rug.

She also discusses the broken bead in Native beadwork that is an act of homage being paid, in a sense, to imperfection; that this is part of life and must be honored. My scar was the error in stitch, the broken bead made in me. I began my life in imperfection. But this imperfection was divine, my scar a lifeline. I pray to be free from a need to be perfect and from the anger at myself when I am not.

Fifteen of us sit on breath stools in a circle. Some stretch their legs, leaning over to touch toes; some sit at the edge, backs straight, hands on knees, eyes closed. Juerg asks us to check in with our breath as we begin class. As I sit quietly sensing my breath, I ask myself, where is my body? The word *dead* wells up. Next I hear, *well, I feel myself breathing, so I must be alive.*

Juerg leads us through a wonderful progression of exercises and in the final segment, we are free to explore movement on our own. I notice that I am responding to each breath in a fresh way, no two body movements alike. I feel "body walls," a term that Juerg has referred to earlier, in front and back—a friendly enclosure.

"I have body walls!" I blurt during the sharing as we rest on our stools.

Juerg nods, smiling with satisfaction.

When I get home and report my discovery to Griffin, she says, "Our lives are going to change."

My lover Griffin and I are kissing and holding each other. I undress, wanting to be close to her body. Before we embrace, she looks at me lying naked. I can't stand being seen, the scar splitting my center. I want to apologize for being damaged goods, for how ugly I am, how she is stuck with me.

"My scar," I cry, upset with myself for interrupting our flow. "I don't, well, I'm dealing with it."

"Let me see it," Griffin offers.

I look down at the series of raised, crooked lines.

"I like it," she says. She counts the stitches, guiding her eyes with her finger. "Twelve."

"There were more inside," I add, "underneath. Why do you like it?" I ask as she covers me with the sheet and pulls me close to her.

"Because it saved you."

Later that night, at an open mic, a man reads from his poem: "Yes, you are scarred, god dammit, and so is everyone else so get over it!" It occurs to me, as I listen raptly in the audience, that maybe all of us are scarred. Perhaps the world is more full of the wounded than I realize, and I am not so different after all. Maybe all the world is like me and I am like all the world.

July 26, my mother, now ninety-one, calls, launching once again into her timeworn description: *you were wrapped in all those tubes, in and out of every opening.* This time, I pressed for a new image.

"Can't you remember anything else? What about my cheeks, my chin, my forehead? What about my nose?"

"Tubes were everywhere," she insisted, "even coming out of your scalp!"

"Try, Mom," I implored. "Think of my face."

For several minutes, she searched quietly inside herself for something she could say. "Your eyes were closed," she said.

I waited for more but nothing came. I imagined two tiny pink shells, pearly and thin, perfect miniatures, like the ones cast onto the shores of the Shrewsbury River at Sandy Hook.

Sponges

Sponges seem to have had a different origin from other members of the animal kingdom and to have traveled a solitary evolutionary route.

—Helena Curtis, *Biology 4th edition*

"I am cherry alive" the little girl sang

—Delmore Schwartz, poem

Sometimes in life we are called upon to do something big. It is a necessary, important thing. At the time, though, it is unwanted, as if doing anything else would be better. As if someone else should do it. But there is no one else. Just you.

Driving home on Interstate 5 from Griffin's brother's funeral in Los Angeles, a week of miracles and heartbreaks in which Max died from blood cancer while on a ventilator, my cell rings. We pull onto a ramp. The police called, my brother tells me, informing him that my mother had 911-ed them three times that week to report a break-in. I call Margaret to check on Mom. "She's flippin' her lid, Wend. You better come." When Griffin and I arrive home, I book a flight to New Jersey.

As the taxi hangs a left from Voorhees Street onto Arthur, my mother's close friend Ray leans out his front door and waves me over. On his living room couch sits my mother, talking nonstop. Her skin is sallow, her hair disheveled, her dress unkempt. I have never seen her like this. Ray tells me that she has knocked the deadbolts and latches out of the front and back doors the night before, thinking that she was locked inside her house and unable to get out.

I walk my mother home, my arm through hers, Ray behind carrying my bags. Inside the house, a heap of metal tools lie on the kitchen table; three holes gape in the back door where the locks and doorknob used to be. In the front door is a disk of air where the deadbolt once resided. It is time to make decisions.

After days of ferrying my mother around to doctors, making order in her house, and getting her back on a three-meal-a-day schedule, I head down to Conant Woods, the park adjacent to the railroad tracks, a sizable acreage of trees through which the Elizabeth River runs. It flows past Conant Estates, a housing tract the building of which, according to my mother, destroyed all the flowering dogwood, and forks at a large pharmaceutical manufacturing plant in the city of Union. When I lived with my parents, I'd come here to chill out when I was upset and needed time to myself. Now, I was back with new issues. Should I move my mother to California or hire someone to help in her home? What about moving back to New Jersey? Could I get a job here? Would Griffin want to move? What about my tenured teaching job at the community college?

As I hike along the trails at Salem, I become preoccupied with memories of the past—me as a confused thirteen-year-old smoking cigarettes, drinking with friends, and making out with my boyfriend, hidden from adult eyes by the trees and brush of these woods. I accept the sadness I feel seeing the despoiled river, riverbank, and flood plain and ask forgiveness for the part I've played in its destruction.

I experience an opening and become aware of my breath. I feel my chest lift and fall. I sense breath in my knees, my elbows, my middle. The earth carries my feet, allowing me to open to trust. The forest comes to life. I notice a particularly wonderful archway of reed-like stalks, providing a yellow ochre canopy over the winding trail. From these slim branches hang delicate, papery three-sided hearts with a single seed at the center, like a tiny dark eye. To my left, land rises, swelling into gentle hills where wild onions grow. At the base of one of these hills, buff-colored grass sprouts with feathery tufts, each supported by a spine composed of tiny, stiff spikes crossed like a row of Xs.

Nature has gone about its business, regardless of the mustard-colored silt at the bottom of a nearby rivulet, the result of the dumping of chemicals; regardless of the eyesore of plastic bottles, wrappers, and packages strewn throughout the flood plain, hanging from branches, smashed into soil or simply lying in the brush; despite an eerie buzzing coming from a strange pair of thick metal posts emerging from the ground just across the river from the huge pharmaceutical plant; and despite a toxic, teal sheen painting the water with an unnatural iridescence. Wherever I look, the secrets of this small stand of woods open to me. Maples and oaks tower overhead, short green and tall buff grasses flourish in the lowland and bromeliad-looking plants sprout from higher ground. Far from being destroyed, the forest is resilient.

Standing on a footbridge, I stare into the flowing water and imagine a small fish swimming in the way that fish do, curving its body in and out. In all the time I spent here as a child and young adult, I have never seen a fish or evidence that one existed. No splash from the quick turn of a tail or a break of the surface by a fish snatching a fly. What type of creatures lived here once upon a time? Could fish live here again? Is there any life in this river now?

Later that evening, my mother surprises me by handing me a black and white photo of Salem Dam along the Elizabeth River, not knowing that I had just returned from roaming downstream from that very place. In the photo, two young women, wearing clothes characteristic of the thirties, sit on the concrete levee, enjoying the pristine view. Thick canopies that cast deep shade tower over a wide river, rushing past banks free of debris. The bushes bordering the banks are lush, shelter for ducklings and protection against erosion. This is the Salem she remembers and loves.

This photo testifies not only to how the river and its environs once thrived, but also how they could do so again. A wonderful thought strikes me: Now that I am bringing myself back from the dead, I can do anything. It is time to bring my mother to California.

I spend the month packing up my mother and her cat, Omega. Griffin finds an apartment for them just down the street from our place, since a trailer on ten acres of dry and rocky land is no place for a mom, and spends weeks decorating and furnishing it. The day that my cousin pulls out of my mother's driveway with my mother and me on our way to the airport goes down as one of the saddest days of my life. I'll never forget Ray walking away unable to face us, and my mother sitting next to me in the back seat, hugging the cat carrier and shaking her head. One week after my fifty-second birthday, my mother, her cat Omega, and I fly into San Francisco International Airport. Griffin meets us at the baggage claim, rushing toward us pushing a baggage cart. Seeing her is one of the happiest moments of my life. We are not alone. We are loved.

The moment that we open the door of her new apartment, a wave first of relief and then thankfulness, washes over me: the brightly painted white walls; the spacious kitchen; the cozy brown and orange sofa. My mother walks swiftly into the living room and plants herself happily on the couch. Thus our new life begins.

After two short weeks of a basically pleasant transition—fixing up her home, going on walks, and setting her up with different services in town— my mother trips on a grate in the street and breaks a pelvic bone. She is admitted to the hospital and we scramble to supervise her care. One morning I'm so stressed that I back the truck into a much more substantial truck as I pull out of my parking space at the hospital. A deep gash bisects the truck's tailgate, but it still works. Oddly, it reminds me of my scar.

The following day on the hospital patio, I happen to see my and Griffin's doctor, Dr. Piper, as she sweeps across the pavement in a light-blue, gauzy blouse, her long blonde hair rippling over her shoulders in soft waves. She chats with patients pushing IV poles on wheels or sunning themselves in wheelchairs, an angel spreading stardust. When she hears why I am there, she offers to attend my mother. I am beyond grateful.

Later that week, I see Dr. Piper, too for back pain. She is an amazing osteopath, a Renaissance physician. Since my mother arrived, I'd alternated between sleeping on blankets on the floor and a box spring. My lower back was killing me. "You know," she says as I lie on the table, "I've met your family. I know your mother now and, of course, I know Griffin, and I see what is going on. Your mother interrupted your aura, you know. She traumatized you with her trauma." She bends my leg and moves it slowly up to my waist. She pushes against my thigh for a minute or so and releases it. She presses again.

I tell her about my operation, how my mother both saved me and blamed me. "Many children survive trauma quite well, you know," she tells me. "When I was two, my aunt ran me over in her car. I was a loved child, and what could have been an awful time was a very wonderful time for me. The other children at the hospital were jealous of the presents that I received from my family and all the time they spent with me there. I was loved," she repeats. "I was so loved. I knew that I was just the most special little person. And I ate it up; I loved being loved that way." She says that she passed through the trauma and bounced right back.

"I was special and I was a burden," I told her. "One minute I was a princess and the next, I was the devil, back and forth."

"Your mother hung onto the trauma, and it's your job now to help your mother let it go before she dies. Tell her, I'm so glad it's over. It's past. Good-bye," she says, waving to the trauma as she sweeps past me and slides her palm under my head, fingers pressing firmly against the cords of my neck. As Dr. Piper works, I become aware of my spine. The symbolism associated with the backbone does not escape me: courage, integrity, stability. The image of a dolphin comes to me—how its long, strong body curves effortlessly, propelling it through water.

Dr. Piper turns serious. "You know, don't you, that you probably didn't receive anesthesia?"

"Yes," I say, surprised by this sudden affirmation of what I'd learned. "I researched this recently." My eyes tear up.

"No anesthesia?" she play-acted. "No problem. She won't remember. She's too little. She doesn't feel anything anyway. She's only a baby, a mere speck. We're the ones who remember," she said, puffing out her chest. She flashes her mischievous eyes on me. My tears turn first to belly-laughter as I imagine those who banked on my forgetting the operation and then joy as I revel in her imp-like presence, basking in her passionate defense of me.

She ends the session with a manipulation that she calls "the Brazilian toehold." She pulls my two pinky toes simultaneously and holds them extended for several minutes. Then the next two toes and the next. She seems to be resetting my nervous system, allowing the juices to flow in a new direction. When she releases my last two toes, it is as if she has cracked open a nugget of amber and laid the ancient mosquito on the counter. She tells me that I've got to stop feeling sorry, stop apologizing for making my mother's life hard, for making her suffer. Sorry, sorry, sorry—the mantra of my life. "Enough already. You have nothing to be sorry for. You never have."

That evening when I get back to my mother's apartment, the door flies open and there stand Griffin and my mother wearing purple party hats, blowing party favors, and waving streamers with HAPPY BIRTHDAY printed in red on white. My mother now leans on a fancy walker with hand breaks and a seat. A luscious chocolate cake waits on the kitchen table. Griffin says I am finally getting the birthday party I missed in the summer when home in New Jersey with Mom. I know what we are really celebrating though. I have grown a backbone. Griffin gives me travel books about France, my mother a writer's treasure box, filled with calligraphy pens and bottles of dark ink. It reminds her, she says, of her mother's writing box. "Women wrote letters back then," my mother explains. "Time to get writing." Little do they know that this is kind of a send-off party, bon voyaging me into my new life.

My mother has long since stopped remembering which day of the week it is, and the day of the month is completely off her radar. This July 26, I choose not to tell my mother the date. I do not want to hear those cobwebbed words—*all those tubes, in and out of everywhere, alien from outer space*—and she does not bring up the subject. I have a better way to mark the day—a massage that Griffin bought me for my birthday. A time to cherish my body. A time to take care of that baby.

A profound understanding of my body comes to me in a workshop given by the founder of breathwork, Ilse Middendorf, who traveled from Germany to teach a class at the Breath Institute in the States. Born in 1910, she worked with many innovative somatic practitioners and in 1965, established the Institute for the Experienced Breath in Berlin. She is a master body worker and her workshop is a precious opportunity. I arrange weekend respite care for Mom to give Griffin and me this chance to work with Ilse, Griffin's first breath teacher.

Ilse, slight with short blonde hair, stands at one end of the room. Her body is so alive and full of breath; every move she makes is vital—graceful and deliberate. Next to her, Greta, a breath teacher in San Francisco, interprets her words from German to English. I love the lilt of Ilse's voice and the softness with which her words emerge. I'd always thought the German language harsh until I heard it from Ilse.

At one point, she gives the direction to do free work—to sense the breath in your body and let it move you wherever it would like. I find myself hunkering down, dwelling mostly in the lower space of my pelvis and legs as if I were prevented from rising. As a toddler, I did not crawl because I was afraid to; my insides might spill out through the scar on my belly. I chose the safer mode—"hitching," as my mother called it, on my butt by digging my heels into the floor and pulling myself forward. I begin to cry in class, feeling immense compassion for myself as a little girl trying to feel at home in the world.

Gradually, as I continue to sense my breath, my movements grow larger. I am a cup-shaped sea creature, a combination of a staghorn coral and a giant sponge, dancing in the currents. My shoulders, usually like clamps pressing down, loosen and begin to float on the ocean of breath, gently rising and falling. I sway, rooted at my base. In the past, I wasn't large enough inside to hold big dreams—the field of marine biology, the ocean, the Ivy League. I couldn't trust enough to let my dreams carry me. I didn't believe that I deserved a big and beautiful life.

In the workshop, I discover a new space within me. I move upward and outward, spiraling up from the lower space, my hands tracing wide curves. I am opening, swaying widely, reaching for more than I ever dared, touching the vast world with my fingertips, inviting it in. *I am the largeness of this world*, my body dances. Ilse shines her gaze on me and speaks. "Dancer," Greta interprets.

I have loved sponges from the moment I saw their single, frail line branching off the phylogenetic tree in my biology textbook. Robust survivors, the sponge with its simple structure has remained basically the same for hundreds of millions of years. Their existence gives me a sense of the rightness of things. How deeply satisfying to think that something could be made right the first time.

Sponges haven't had to deal with stomachs. For them, a simple digestive system is the way to go, no mouth or esophagus necessary. Food is drawn into the body through external pores that lead into canals that direct the water, hence nourishment, throughout the organism. I wonder if sponges know how lucky they are to be coated with a special substance to prevent the plugging of pores.

In the simplest, bulb-shaped sponges, water is channeled into a central cavity, where cells lining the cavity engulf food and transfer it to other types of cells where further digestion occurs. Finally, the water exits from a single osculum, or large pore. Larger sponges, while using this same type of system, have internal walls that fold, as do human stomachs, thus increasing surface area for digestion. The most complex sponges are composed of large internal chambers. A basic filtration system though has served sponges well for millions of years. Flow is their specialty.

For centuries, sponges eluded classification. In the days of the Greeks, they were called plants though Aristotle claimed that they were zoophytes or "animal-plants." In the 1700s, an English scientist observed that certain cells caused water currents to flow through the organisms, a phenomenon more characteristic of a plant. They were still considered, however, zoophytes. Confusion continued into the 1900s when it was decided that sponges are part of the animal kingdom, but because their origin is somewhat unique, they are considered a subkingdom unto themselves: parazoa, meaning bordering or beside animals. Sponges are now classified as phylum Porifera, the many-holed ones.

Sponges have persisted under duress with no means of fighting back—they are sessile and can't escape, and do not have claws, barbs, or poison. They resist bacterial infection, are distasteful to fish and most other marine creatures, and are able to regenerate themselves after subjection to sun and air. Completely dried out, sponges come alive again when in contact with water. Cells within the organism, called gemmules, reactivate, enabling growth to continue. Sponges hold the power to raise themselves from the dead. In this way, I am like them.

I lie wrapped in warm blankets under the soft, yellow light of shaded lamps, Juerg sitting by my side and talking quietly after a one-on-one session. A soft, jelly-like place exists inside me just below my sternum near my solar plexus and under the scar on my abdomen, where the breath rises and falls effortlessly—a breathbeat at the center of my body that I feel slowly pulsing. I am not controlling it. It is a part of myself of which I have just become aware—a sort of island at the center of my being. The integrity of what he calls the core, my beingness or my source, was not violated, not affected by the operation. "The surface was altered," he says, "yes, the scar is evidence of this. Only the surface though." With his words, a deep fear I hadn't known I had, that some unnamable essential part of me had been compromised, lifted.

I don't need to try so hard to make things happen in my life, Juerg tells me; I can "allow" them. "The core is there, and you can trust." I understand that the operation has not touched my center, my strength. Breath is coming and going on its own. My core is alive. I can trust my body. Sitting up, I notice the cherry wood carving of a dolphin arcing in its leap from the sea. *Has that always been there in the corner?* I wonder.

In the breath class following this private work, a new sense of myself melds into my understanding. When Juerg gives the direction to do free work, breath movement lifts my arms and then lowers them. The body of breath extends, radiating out like the walls of a sponge into the surrounding waters so that I feel larger; I take up more space. That I am anchored to my core, my place in the sand, allows me to grow wider. Shafts of soft green and turquoise light fall around me. Effortlessly, my arms reach out wider, offering themselves to the sun-lit currents. I am an invitation open to where my breath is taking me.

In my 52ⁿᵈ year, I am beginning to understand the complexities of evolution. Altruism, according to biologist Loren Eiseley, is a force in nature that determines survival and, therefore, has its own validity in natural selection. In his book *The Starthrower*, he discusses a profound encounter, which opened his eyes to this phenomenon. Up at five a.m. one day and walking on the beach, he saw a man whom he subsequently referred to as the Starthrower. Each day, Eiseley learned, this man rose before dawn so that he could scour the beach before others arrived. He would do this in order to save those starfish that had been stranded by the tide, throwing them back into the ocean as I had done as a girl with the upended horseshoe crabs. In this way, Eiseley claims, altruism influences the survival of a species.

Anthropologist Jane Goodall also pays homage to the power of altruism with regard to species' viability. She discovered in her observation of chimps that the fight or flight mode is only a part of what informs the behavior of an animal: "From an evolutionary perspective, individuals form very close family bonds first. For a mother or older brother to be compassionate and caring to the infants, for example, benefits the family—makes it stronger, more members survive . . . When a member of the group is altruistic toward another member who is suffering, it's beneficial to the group as a whole . . . So our altruism probably extended as our brains became more complex." Altruism, a determining factor of evolution, has shaped our world. It certainly has molded mine.

My scar is a mark of altruism. Those who helped to save me recognized my parents' plight and, motivated by compassion, took action to alleviate suffering. This humanitarian effort initiated a series of events: Dr. Constad, diagnosing the problem; a surgeon summoned from New York City; nurses monitoring my progress; my parents devoted to my recovery; my aunt and uncle caring for my brother. The healed over stitches are like so many arms reaching out. The scar is a mark of love.

Life is a process of playing with patterns: unraveling those that no longer serve us and reweaving the strands into ones that do. It's not about throwing away or excising anything. It's about understanding, forgiving, and allowing reorganization from the inside out, trusting things will come out alright. More than alright; even beautiful. Many types of starfish can create a new, fully functioning arm from a damaged one. Though the organism's wholeness has been compromised, it regenerates a new self. An old pattern, no matter how intricately woven, can be undone and rewoven into the whole. Our wounds teach us how to heal. Our wounds teach us how to grow.

The way I view the world is changing. One night after breath class, as I walk along under a clear sky, the stars shining crisply white in contrast to the deep ultramarine blue, a particular cloud catches my attention: elongate, prone, three connected puffs—head, body and legs. *Dead baby*, I think. This conclusion does not sit well with me. Am I seeing what is really there?

As I study the cloud further, I realize it is fresh and white, the "chest" even a bit fluffy, and the head held up at a slight angle. This observation matches my inner feeling more closely. The night sky is alive and charged with energy—the clouds, the sky, trees, stars, moon hidden behind the clouds, light breaking through. I notice that my lips are pressed together into what my mother calls a "buttermilk grin," suppressing the overwhelming joy I feel. I have photos of me as a girl grinning like that. Even during my happiest moments, my jaw muscles clamped down. If I burst with happiness, my stitches would burst, too. But now the power of joy wins out. I break into a smile, run down the street, and reach my arms up to the clouds, twirling in circles. *The baby is alive, and so am I!*

At a breath workshop led by Griffin outside of Sacramento, one of the participants, a naturopathic doctor, asks me whether I am going to become a breath practitioner. I tell her no, that breathwork gave me a vehicle to heal from the trauma of an operation I underwent at three weeks old. Her eyebrows rise in curiosity, so I continue. "I realize that my body is not my enemy. I ran away from it; it was too dangerous to be in. Breathwork enabled me to find my way back."

"You know," she replies, "that's similar to what I tell my patients. If we aren't present in our homes, we are vulnerable to burglars. If we are not present in our bodies, disease can enter."

My mother can no longer live in the apartment. We had no idea how much dementia had claimed her until the night Griffin was awoken by some commotion in the living room at two in the morning. Griffin and I had been taking turns sleeping over my mother's while she was getting used to the new apartment.

"Mom," Griffin said, "where are you going?" My mother was fully clothed and her purse hung from her arm.

"To the bank. You two won't take me, so I'm going on my own. I want my money and you two have been pilfering from me."

"Mom, it's two o'clock in the morning. The bank isn't even open."

"Oh, yes it is, sister. I know your game." She turned back to fiddling with the deadbolt.

When Griffin approached her and she raised her cane, a turning point had been reached.

Griffin calls me, crying into the phone, "I just can't do this!" I completely understood. Taking care of my mother was beyond taxing. A few days before, Griffin had been out in the back yard watering some plants before driving my mother to day care when, unbeknownst to her, my mother quietly opened the front door and left. Griffin found her several blocks away on Highway 193, thumbing a ride. A car pulled up just as Griffin caught up with my mother. Furious, my mother hurried across the street (of course, she hadn't taken her walker) and then proceeded to evade Griffin for the next two hours.

Time for respite care—for us and for my mother. We pack her up for a week's stay at Sunshine, a small care place for elders run by a lovely woman named Ruth. She has cared for my mother before and one of the caregivers there, Carmella, has taken a special liking to my mother. We say good-byes at the front door, which fortunately locks when it shuts.

∾∾∾

In another session with Dr. Piper, she places her hands under my head and presses her fingers into my neck as she speaks to me in a soft voice. "Do you know about Kali, the compassionate goddess? We often think of compassion as mushy or soft, but Kali carries a sword. She is focused and gets things done." She folds one of my legs over the other. "How's that?"

"Good."

"You probably never got to experience the body as comfort," she says as she holds my leg in position. "When there's pain, the brain shuts off certain neurotransmitters. It shuts down cells. The brain isolates you from the painful part of the body. Until you end the isolation of this body part, the immune system will not be fully available to this area, and you will be subject to disease."

"You know, I finally realized that my stomach is good!"

She smiles. "I have a prescription for you, young lady. Get a bottle of sesame oil. Your skin needs omega-3. Rub it all over. Finish out the bottle. Start with your stomach, radiate out. Bodies need touching. Do this yourself. As you massage the oil in, say to yourself, *I am whole, I am whole.*"

As directed, after a hot shower, I rub myself with oil. I feel a little weird;

I'm not used to pampering. Touching myself without tension is a challenge. I do as told, though, telling myself I am whole. I believe it some of the time and that's when the massaging feels good. When my fingers feel the bumps of my scar, I notice that I am holding my breath. As usual, I'm afraid I'll explode. Realizing this, I allow breath into my middle space. Breath fills my belly. What relief!

Sesame oil is thick, so I lie back to let it soak in. I remember a fish that lives permanently inside the Venus flower basket, a deep-water "glass" sponge whose walls are formed by spicules of silica. When the fish is small, it comes and goes as it pleases. But as the fish grows, it becomes too large to leave its enclosure. From then on, the fish and the sponge live together. How limiting, I had once thought—to be imprisoned one's whole life inside the body of another organism.

Lying there with a light blanket pulled up over my naked, glistening body, I realize how beautiful their bonding actually is. The fish cleans parasites from the sponge, and the body of the sponge serves as protection for the fish. Their association brings stability, harmony itself as they float in the cold ocean, a world of their own making—body and spirit living in joyous exchange. My scar and I living symbiotically, the biology of understanding between us.

During this time, I had one of the most powerful dreams of my life: me as a grinning baby, brandishing five swords in each hand. Not puny knives but large, heavy swords with sharp, wide blades. My eyes shone. I was slicing, swinging the swords over my head. Anyone who came near, slash! I was a cowgirl spinning my deadly lariats, Kali with multiple arms slicing everything in my path. I was a sword girl, a deadly baby, dangerous, thrilled with my power. No one dared come near. Everyone was terrified. I was a caricature of a Whirling Dervish, my knives spinning so fast, they blurred. My fists bulged with blades, and I smiled devilishly. I had never been happier.

Practicing breathwork one day, I follow my cycle – inhale, exhale, pause – and discover tension crowding my breath at the end of exhale. The image of a gaping maw appears in my head—a white shark with a huge circle of jagged, sharp teeth. It's my swollen renegade stomach, hell-bent on destroying my life. My mother's fear of my illness returning, which I took on, has lived inside of me all these years, limiting my every breath.

Amazed at the clarity with which I suddenly see this creature, this manifestation of my terror, I take out red clay from the trailer storage shelf and sculpt it. Under the old, smooth bark of the manzanita tree, I shape the teeth and powerful jaw. The body of the shark is small—it's the enormous mouth I'm consumed by. I set the clay sculpture on the table still in shock that something so dangerous could have lived inside me, threatening the waters for decades without my knowing.

As a child, I didn't have the tools to deal with this invader, nor did my parents, nor the professionals around me. Growing up, I tried to kill it— alcohol, smoke, food gorges, food deprivation, overdoses of pills, cutting— yet the white shark never budged. A deeper aspect of my past obsession with suicide became clear: I was trying to kill the creature inside that had taken over, separating me from my authentic self.

Continuing the exploration of my breath cycle, I notice that I hold back from completing exhale. Instead of pausing, I jump right to inhale. Each time, I skip the pause, that delicate place of peace. There's a connection between the gaping maw and this lack of pause. The creature lurks between breaths, swallowing up the resting place where I might find balance. This missing pause disrupts my ability to say "yes" and "no" to what life offers. I lack boundaries, definition. At the end of exhale as I leap over my pause to inhale, I don't give my real self a safe place to be. The creature swallows it. My breath is still running away from my stomach though it's been healed for fifty years.

During breath class with Juerg, I face my fear of the shark. In an exercise called "small steps," in which we sense breath as we walk, I become especially aware of the movement of breath in my back between my shoulder blades. As I approach a picture on the wall, I see an image of the gaping mouth within swirls of muted color, waiting to swallow me. I know that it is a projection of what I am dealing with inside, yet still, I am afraid.

Suddenly, I feel propelled by a new force of breath pushing me forward, providing the power to move. It is as if I am being shoved from behind. Face to face with the gaping maw, it dissolves into beige blandness. The white shark, once confronted, is not real. Like in the movie *The Wizard of Oz*, the thing one fears is not in itself powerful. The power that one gives it makes it dangerous.

All my life, I lived a fantasy. There was no invader who could take my life. I would have no "trouble" in my fifties, as my mother had worried about and my pediatrician, Dr. Constad, was very concerned about—so much so that he checked for that swelling in my abdomen until I was twelve! So was my whole life a waste, one big exercise in imagination run wild? No, because the fear was real. The terror was palpable.

Had I pursued marine biology in an unconscious effort to confront this shark? Perhaps I studied life, "bio-", in an attempt to conquer death. By studying biology, I was trying to save myself.

I did not become a marine biologist. Blame it on lack of confidence; poor math skills; corrupt scientists; sexism in science; confusion about which area to specialize in; lack of vision and determination; cold turkey withdrawal from prescription Valium at Barnard and the resulting suicide attempt; the *bad baby* mantra. The fact that I just didn't believe I was capable of anything grand. Blame it on my subconscious motivation for choosing a biology major in the first place. Frankly, I had no more control over my life than those sea creatures; strong currents tossed us both. They, however, had adapted more successfully. After all, they were simply themselves. And in growing up, I was far from simply being me.

As a teenager, I wanted to be like Jacques Cousteau and crew, sailing around the globe and exploring the underwater world, one month studying coral in the Red Sea, another month stingrays or octopuses off the coast of California. In the field of science though, I always ended up behind a machine, hitched to sophisticated technology: the atomic adsorption spectrophotometer; the ultrasonic cell sonifier; the Millipore filter. Science is all about measurement, but I leaned toward using a different ruler.

I wanted to observe, marvel, be surprised. Measuring, graphing, and comparing maimed the mystery. To do biology in the '70s, though, quantification was the key to the kingdom. Even my favorite marine biologist besides Rachel Carson, Dr. Eugenie Clark, who studied, among other subjects, eels in the Red Sea and whom I admire for her poetic and thoughtful observations, had to mark out the underwater territory with a precise grid, using poles and rope. She measured the presence of snakes per square foot, recorded increases and decreases in population, noted changes in the flora and fauna, and monitored water chemistry levels for oxygen, nitrogen, nitrates, sulfates, sodium, and magnesium. She created graphs, compared percentages. She did the math. Cousteau and team also relied on state of the art equipment, their research vessels always equipped with the most advanced systems.

Maybe I should have lived in an earlier era. Perhaps a career as an 18th century naturalist would have best suited me, writing copious field notes while perched atop a hummock, not merely noting the numeral "1" for cumulus clouds, "2" for stratus, or "3" for nimbus, but an entry more like this: *The clouds pile high today, thick ice cream sundaes, mounds of vanilla. Turquoise sky. Moisture encloses me with its sticky tendrils. The wind puffs, gentle, warm and unpredictable, grasses bending gracefully to its will.* Yes, this is how I would have liked to have done science.

〜〜〜

My mother is now part of a community for elders with dementia and Alzheimer's, what is called a memory care facility. It's as homey as a place like this can be; she has her own room with wood furniture, her own bathroom, and a view of greenery out her window. The staff is loving and tries hard to keep her busy. They say, "She keeps us laughing." She is ninety-five, and because she is recovering from a hip break, sits most days in a wheelchair. The beloved director is leaving at the end of the month, though, so Griffin and I are looking for a house to buy in which the three of us can live.

When I visit her, we look at photos or page through picture books about animals. Once she asks, "So what have you been doing?"

"I'm finishing a book about my operation."

"What? You had an operation?" She looks puzzled.

"When I was a baby."

"You did?" she asks, eyes widening. "What happened?"

"My food was blocked and I couldn't digest it."

"Well, for pity's sake. I have my problems, too, ya know," she says, pointing to her black cat, lying on her pillow. "This kitty here, I couldn't find her, but here she is on the bed."

"Good—that's nice."

"Getting back to what you said—do you still have problems?"

"No."

"Well, you've carried it all those years," she says, straightening her shoulders and nodding.

"Sure did!"

We laugh.

∽∽∽

As I water the melons in my garden, an image of a healthy stomach comes to mind: a round organ, opalescent pink. It has a smiling mouth and two tiny sparkling eyes. This stomach has been loyal and healthy since the operation and is not a ruthless, red monster with huge, sharp teeth.

I realize how much my stomach has done for me all these years. How faithfully it digests my food and keeps me alive and awash with nutrients. I have given my stomach a bad rap, made it into some frightening predator that could kill me on a whim. I kept my breath away, harboring it shallowly in my lungs, psychically excising the monster tummy from my life. Now it is time to let *breath come and go on its own*, in the words of Juerg. Time to let my stomach be. To say, I am my stomach and my stomach is me.

Stomachs are pouches with openings, valves directing the flow of solution. Sponges too are purse-like—bags with holes, seawater flowing in and out. Stomachs are organs; sponges are organ-like. Both have folds inside that increase the surface area, enabling greater absorption. Stomachs live in the darkness of the body's interior as sponges make their home in the dim depths of the sea. Both are somewhat comical to me, begging for a squeeze.

Breathwork has become a daily practice. Every morning sitting on my breath stool, I feel the support of the earth, alert for insights. The latest: *breathing makes bellies rise and fall. It's just what happens.* If I allow breath to expand my belly, without pushing or pulling in any way, I feel my sitz bones and pelvic floor expand. Amazing that I can sense inhale all the way into the pelvic girdle. Does my breath also expand the sacrum so that the bones of the pelvis swing wide? Yes. All moves within. Breathing massages the body internally, maintaining health. Everything inside of us expands and retracts in a harmonious rhythm—the dance of breath.

Now my life hinges on allowing breath into the places from which it was banished. Joy is my goal now, the fullness of experience. A large barrel sponge taking up its rightful space in a warm-water sea.

Behind our trailer, I watch the full moon rise over the ridge, an amber giant, magnified as it is still close to the horizon. *A belly*, I think. I face the moon squarely, place my hands over my scar, and allow my breath to come and go on its own. My breath is gentle and comforting and fills my body with a feeling of vitality and wholeness. I feel round and wide and beautiful. The black immensity of night holds me. I am breathing the moon. Griffin comes up from behind, puts her arms around my belly and pulls me close. We are breathing the moon. I lean my head back on her shoulder.

It's not that I won't feel the terror again. In fact, every morning when I sit down to meditate, I notice that I still restrict my breath. I reassure myself: *You are safe. You are worthy. You are whole.* My body relaxes and when it locks up again, I comfort myself. Healing is a process. I don't know whether there is an end point. One thing I know with certainty—I am coming home to my body.

Epilogue

These days, pyloric stenosis, medically known as Infantile or Congenital Hypertrophic Pyloric Stenosis (CHPS), is familiar to pediatricians, and the recognition of it is more routine. In urban areas, the surgery is often either a Laparoscopy, Minimal Access Surgery [MIS] or Umbilical Pyloromyotomy, in which the scar is less of an issue. The parents have been by the baby's side continuously in the hospital, except for the surgery, and the baby is typically released from the hospital in a few days with an excellent prognosis.

Autobiography of a Sea Creature depicts my actual experience in the 1950s when the diagnosis was not common and the operation risky. Infant surgery was not routine and the use of anesthesia for babies was not the norm. Infants were often paralyzed with a drug, conscious during surgery. In those days, infants were isolated from their mothers and other family members and sequestered in sterile rooms, no visitors allowed.

Long after my surgery was over, its repercussions continued to resound throughout my life. In many adults' lives, the trauma of infant surgery is still an issue even if they've healed completely as babies and the physical condition that required surgery has long since resolved itself. Depression and emotional disturbance plagued me for many years. How ironic that a baby is operated on to save his or her life and as an adult, this person may kill him or herself because coming to terms with issues the early surgery presents has not been possible.

Many thousands have survived pyloric stenosis. It is one of the most common infant illnesses. Tens of thousands of infants who are now adults have survived surgery without anesthetic. What types of lives are they living?

How have they coped? Since the surgery, I have suffered from depression. I have suffered from Post Traumatic Stress Disorder, or PTSD. Treatment early on for PTSD would have enabled me to have lived an entirely different life, one in which my symptoms would have been recognized, and I could have received help and relief. As we have only recently understood trauma and PTSD, and are still learning about it, many survivors of infant surgery without anesthetic are still struggling to negotiate the early trauma in their lives. How many others besides myself have experienced debilitating self-hatred and depression? My hope is that this book provides insight into the issues that surround early surgery and that society will better learn to cope with affected individuals and their families.

I am hopeful, too, that we will begin to think more creatively about how depression and other mental disturbances develop and are treated. We would do well to consider what Dr. Frederick C. Robbins called "The Long View" in a speech addressing the Society for Pediatric Research in 1962. Though he wrote the following statement over fifty years ago referring to infectious disease, his words are also relevant to the subject of infant surgery: "We are entering a new era in which we are facing the need for relating occurrences that are separated, not by days, weeks, or months, but by years . . . [We] must consider the long-term consequences of a variety of kinds of incidents, many of which may now be considered benign and unimportant." In the long view, the clue to the cure of many mental disturbances and imbalances may be in the stories of the individuals themselves, individuals all of whom carry the capacity of coming home to their bodies.

We must do more to help sick or injured infants heal from the psychological and spiritual anguish that can result from early technological intervention. Everything possible must be done to aid the infant in growing into an adult who feels that his or her surgery or intervention was worthwhile and that his or her life was better saved than not. The community—the families and friends of the infants who will undergo a life-threatening condition in their early months and the institutions that support them, such as schools, hospitals, and places of worship—must relieve the suffering, not prolong it. Counselors, psychiatrists, health professionals, doctors, teachers, and spiritual and religious advisers need to be trained to interface with these children in a beneficial way. Otherwise, we fall short of the positive outcome that we had hoped for in the first place when the child was saved.

Afterword

by Jan Osborn, PhD, RN, MFT

Wendy came to me, in part, because she was seeing herself respond in relationships in ways she didn't like but could not seem to change. At that point, Wendy and her wife had been together over thirty years and though Wendy had worked hard and achieved success with her previous therapist, Middendorf Breathwork, and in couples counseling over the years, many of her self-protective behaviors were still active.

I have worked with trauma for decades. While I had done years of trauma therapy utilizing systems theory, experiential techniques, narrative therapy and parts work, it was the addition of EMDR (Eye Movement Desensitization and Reintegration) that was a game changer for me and therefore, my clients.

I don't think either Wendy or I could have imagined the profundity of the journey we were going to embark on together. Assisting someone on their healing journey from trauma is perhaps one of the most intimate experiences a person can have with another where exploring the deepest, darkest fears and vulnerabilities that one has spent a lifetime hiding and protecting are shared with another. And when you are that other, it is a deep honor. It is a present to be unwrapped bit by bit, revealing just enough to move forward without exposing the whole gift at once. You also know that you need to hold it firmly so as not to drop it, causing further injury, but not so tightly that it cannot reveal itself.

There is something very unique about working with infant trauma. When adults come to therapy, they have memories, words, and words about the words. When someone comes in with infant trauma however, the work is with the body, before words, and well before words about the words. When Wendy first came in, on a certain level, a younger, more distant level, she didn't know she had a body. She knew, though, on so many levels that the body was the problem. Her body was "broken into" when she was an infant, with no relief from the pain, as it was believed at that time that infants couldn't feel pain. And, as can happen with early trauma, the adult words about it in the form of beliefs became her beliefs.

When Wendy initially came to me, she lived in her body in a very contracted way, and her beliefs about life reflected this contraction. This is not uncommon for those who've experienced trauma prior to language development, and because there are no words, those with histories of infant trauma are often greatly misunderstood. The way they live in the world doesn't make sense to others: the "overreaction," constant worry and hypervigilance, sometimes with a persistent feeling of impending doom, anxiety, sometimes including panic, rigidity of body and approach to life, negative outlook, depression, with or without suicidal ideation and/ or attempts, lack of trust and need for control, which causes them to be described as difficult, overemotional, rigid, cold. They are often seen as mentally ill rather than traumatized and wounded. To those of us who understand, these traits make perfect sense, albeit traumatic sense. These are very common signs that trauma has occurred earlier in life and that the person is experiencing wounding in the form of Post Traumatic Stress Disorder (PTSD), which truly is a normal response to an abnormal experience. Some of the behaviors that trauma survivors experience are efforts at protection while others are an attempt at mastery. Wendy, for example, became an advocate for those who had experienced infant surgery without anesthesia.

And then, there are those behaviors that are specific to the circumstances of the trauma and to the adult stories about the trauma that then become the survivors' stories, or the stories they live in reaction to. Thus, in addition to the way the body contracts in reaction to, in Wendy's case, the "break in" of the body, there are deep-seated beliefs that form based on the beliefs of the adults around them. Wendy believed that she was a burden because her mother often talked about how difficult the surgery had been for her. Wendy also believed that if she cried or even breathed too deeply, her body would break open, her insides would fall out, and she would die. Her mother was afraid to hold her, so her touch was of no comfort. As a girl she describes what she referred to as "a deep somatic freeze." She would hold her breath for as long as she could, hold her body as rigidly as she could, in an attempt to determine if she was alive or dead and to control the pain that was long since over.

Some of these carried into adulthood, not necessarily on a conscious level. She continued to have an unsureness as to whether she was alive or dead. The way this showed up in her present was that her body would lock up, she would grind her teeth, and her breath would become very shallow. She explained that her own body would decide that it was dangerous to itself before she was even quite awake, with low-grade constant tension and holding of the breath. She was terrified that she didn't have a self, and at the same time, that her self was sick and repulsive, broken, unworthy, unlovable, and didn't belong anywhere. She also believed that she had to do great things to make up for her brokenness. She looked to relationships for rescue, and at the same time, found it very difficult to let in positive attention. Further, she equated love with excessive worry and over-caretaking. And then, what is also common among survivors of trauma is the lack of ability to trust anyone and the anger, a deep-seated rage that you have been harmed, abused, wronged, and there were people to blame for this.

There is also a natural ability of children that Buddhists refer to as "beginner's mind," before all the beliefs of the adults get fully entrenched in young minds. This is the time when they seem to connect with other beings, such as pets, trees, insects, and sea creatures. When there's been trauma and resultant attachment injury, children can identify quite strongly with these other beings. As a little girl, Wendy found her attachment in the sea creatures and her curiosity about them. She wanted to know everything about them, including how their bodies worked, leading her to want to be a scientist, specifically a marine biologist. This too was a reaction of mastery. If she could figure out how they worked, just maybe she could figure out how she worked. Unfortunately, the impact of her early trauma would make it impossible for her to obtain this dream.

The nervous system holds all of this like a computer memory storage. Trauma in childhood leads to reactions and adaptations which impact one's view of self, others and the world and thus, their responses to them. This way of being in the world gets carried into each stage of life because the nervous system continues to detect danger. This, in turn, can tremendously impact relationships with others. The good news about the relational reactions is that they are often directly linked to the trauma. Thus, by exploring patterns of what takes the nervous system out of its safe, balanced place and sends it into fight, flight, or freeze, or what Wendy and I affectionately called flopping, in response to a current situation, we can uncover the links to traumatic events, reactions and beliefs that are locked into the nervous system and change them. Techniques, such as mindfulness and breathing exercises, can help regulate the nervous system response once triggered, thus, managing the reactions. Healing the trauma and shifting child beliefs to beliefs from an adult perspective with trauma therapies, such as EMDR, or Eye Movement Desensitization and Reintegration, allows for the nervous system reaction to be much more regulated, or not even happen in the first place.

EMDR, developed by Francine Shapiro, PhD, in the late 1980s, is a widely researched, evidence-based approach to trauma. It stimulates the brain in ways that lead it to process unhealed memories leading to a natural restoration and adaptive resolution of the nervous system's fight, flight, freeze response. Traumatic events often resolve on their own; however, when they are locked in the nervous system, the mind and body will react as if anything that resembles the original trauma in current life is a serious danger. Thus, people living with unresolved traumatic events will react as if minor events are dangerous. The process of EMDR reduces the vividness of the memory almost as if it's fading. Clients will often say things like, "It's still there but it feels sort of distant." This distance allows the nervous system to no longer act as if it is in danger in the present, thus, trauma reactions are reduced.

This profound process is actually simple. While the client maintains a dual focus on the traumatic event and body stimulation, such as eye movement, connections are made between the physical body and mind, improving cognition. Obviously, in the case of infant trauma, the memory itself may not be present. Thus, focusing on the other areas becomes prominent, such as entrenched, negative core beliefs.

Wendy expressed that she had intense reactions to stimuli she did not understand. In working with preverbal trauma, it is precisely these reactions that give us clues as to what things we need to target in EMDR. With an adult trauma, we can process the incident itself. We look at the event, the feelings around the event, the belief about the event, and also the body's reaction to the event while using EMDR. With infant trauma, we need to start with the body and the beliefs that others told us about the event. Thus, Wendy and I spent countless hours in EMDR sessions on the contraction in her body. What was the held breath trying to tell us? Why was there such an aversion to bright lights or people wearing masks? From there, we could look at how this contracted body reflected contractions in her daily life, like the fear of getting lost on a trip or of being too vulnerable with her partner.

Ultimately, she came to believe that she and her body were one. She no longer believed that her body would pop open or that a good, deep breath would kill her. She believed that she was worth saving, living, and loving.

Her body softened, her trust increased, she had compassion for her mother, and she stopped feeling that she was a burden. She even came so far as to say that having feelings was fabulous, even the terrifying ones, like panic. She came to believe that connection with others was of primary importance and was able to accept help and love from others when she was diagnosed with bladder cancer and her body was under attack again, a disease she was able to heal from completely. She also came to know that love is not worry and that she had to give up the relationship to the trauma to have a relationship with herself, her partner, and her ideals. She came to see herself as a baby being hugged by the universe, joyous and free, supported to be herself. She also felt a conscious connection with her young self every day, who is worthwhile and belongs in this world as a wonderful person, whole, complete, and woundless. She said, "For the first time in life I am glad to be alive without question."

Through the course of our time together, she came to realize that she is the sea creatures and is to be cherished as she cherished them. She said, "I wanted to help my peeps, the sea creatures, and ended up helping this strange human species instead."

Jan Osborn, PhD, RN, MFT

Jan Osborn has a bachelor's in nursing, master's and PhD in Marriage and Family Therapy from Syracuse University. She taught Marriage and Family Therapy at Northwestern University in Chicago, California State University, Sacramento, and Alliant International University. She has worked with trauma recovery for over thirty years. Prior to becoming a marriage and family therapist, she worked as a nurse, specializing in hospice and AIDS work. She has also been a practitioner of mindfulness meditation for 35 years.

Acknowledgments

Mom, who claimed she was a "poet and didn't know it," a writer and lifelong voracious reader who teamed up with my dad to save me after my surgery at one-month-young.

Fred Vanderbom for blogging faithfully alongside me for over a decade, co-creating a community of people who care deeply about the trauma of infant surgery without anesthesia and for affirming our own experiences.

Robin Martin of Two Songbirds Press for her wise counsel and exemplary skill on the final edit of this book.

Red Fox Poets Underground Poetry Collective of the Sierra Foothills, Placerville, California for nourishing my lyric voice, strengthening my confidence, and cultivating deep friendships: Irene Lipshin, Brigit Truex, Moira Magneson, Kate Wells, Taylor Graham, Lara Gularte, Carol Lynn Stevenson Grellas, Jen Vernon, Patricia Caspers, and Carol Louise Moon.

Dr. Marilyn Chandler McEntyre for introducing me to the study of medical humanities and nourishing my writer's voice.

Dr. David Watts and Dr. Joan Baranow for convening the Writing the Medical Experience conferences those many years and creating a vibrant, loving community of talented writers interested in the intersection of medicine and literature.

Trauma experts who taught me how to understand what happened to me as a baby and its effect on me as I grew: Dr. Peter Levine, Dr. Bessel van der Kolk, Dr. Robert Scaer, Dr. Daniel J. Siegel, Dr. Stephen Porges, Dr. Judith Herman, Dr. Bruce Perry, Dr. Lenore Terr, Dr. Gabor Mate, Dr. Louis Tinnin, and Dr. Linda Gantt.

Dr. Jan Osborn, therapist and EMDR practitioner extraordinaire, who helped me bring more calm to my nervous system and who introduced me to the teachings of Buddhist teacher Thich Nhat Hanh.

Juerg Roffler, founder of MIBE, Middendorf Institute for Breathexperience, Berkeley, California and co-founder of MIBE Berlin, who taught me how my body was wounded from infant surgery and how it could heal.

Manuscript readers who encouraged me and supercharged my spirit: Judy Wells, Jean Anne Zollars, Robert Clover Johnson, and Harriet Harstoll.

Roey Shmool, who created a film featuring stories about life in the aftermath of infant surgery without anesthesia and the lives of parents of newborns who were ill and did not receive pain control for their surgeries. *Cutdown: Infant Surgery without Anesthesia* is available on YouTube: (https://youtu.be/PX6LNHUX7zo)

Jolene Philo whose writings on her blog A Different Dream helped affirm my understanding about PTSD in the aftermath of infant surgery without anesthesia.

Susan Ito, Audrey Ferber, and Leanna James Blackwell, my Mills College MFA grad school buddies, whose love and writing feedback sustained me for many years and whose friendships continue to nourish.

Susan Griffin for hearing and encouraging the earliest drafts of this book.

Susan Chernilo for encouraging my expression of self through writing as I suffered with depression and for extending her friendship during my darkest of times.

Close friends Sheila O'Rourke and Renee Chavez for always believing in my writing, this project, and me.

Mary Fifield for loving, monthly support and for keeping me committed to expressing my authentic voice and getting my words out into the world.

Carol Imani for her caring and deep listening in drawing out my thoughts in the process of writing the book proposal.

Editor Brian Dolan for encouraging me in submitting the manuscript to University of California Health Humanities Press and his sublime patience and expertise in shepherding this book to final product.

Griffin Toffler, my precious companion of forty-one years, wife of thirteen years, who has been my most potent editor and nourisher of my creative spirit.

References

Horseshoe Crabs

Rudloe, Anne and Jack. "The Changeless Horseshoe Crab." *National Geographic* April 1981: 562–572. Print.

The Intertidal Zone

National Geographic Society. *The Ocean Realm*. Washington, D.C.: National Geographic Society, 1978. Print.

Nigricans

National Geographic Society. *The Ocean Realm*. Washington, D.C.: National Geographic Society, 1978. Print.

Divine Imperfection

Anand, K. J. S., and P. R. Hickey. "Pain and its Effects in the Human Neonate and Fetus." *New England Journal of Medicine* 317.21 (1987): 1321–1329. Print.

Benson, Dr. Clifford. "Infantile Pyloric Stenosis: Historical Aspects and Current Surgical Concepts." *Progress in Pediatric Surgery*, 1970. 1: 63–88. Print.

Chamberlain, David B. "Babies Don't Feel Pain." *Cyborg Babies: From Techno Sex to Techno Tots*. Eds. Robbie Davis-Floyd and Joseph Dumit. New

York: Routledge, 1998: 168–189. Print.

Cook-Sather, Scott D. et al. "A Comparison of Awake Versus Paralyzed Tracheal Intubation for Infants with Pyloric Stenosis." *Pediatric Anesthesia,* 86 (1998): 945–951. Print.

Solnit and Green. "Reactions to the Threatened Loss of a Child: A Vulnerable Child Syndrome." *Pediatrics.* July, 1964: 58–66. Print.

Sponges

Curtis, Helena. *Biology, 4th edition.* New York: Worth Publishers, 1983. Print.

Hunt, Scott A. *The Future of Peace.* San Francisco: HarperCollins Publishers, Inc., 2002. Print.

The Illustrated Encyclopedia of the Animal Kingdom. New York: Grolier, 1971. Print.

National Geographic Society. *The Ocean Realm.* Washington, D.C.: National Geographic Society, 1978. Print.

Epilogue

Robbins, Frederick C. "The Long View." *American Journal of the Diseases of Children,* 104: Nov. (1962): 499–503. Print.

www.ingramcontent.com/pod-product-compliance
Lightning Source LLC
Chambersburg PA
CBHW052133270326
41930CB00012B/2866